THE
POWER
OF
RESTORATIVE
SLEEP

IT IS NOT JUST **IF** YOU SLEEP -
BUT **HOW** YOU SLEEP THAT MATTERS!

Debra J. Stultz M.D.

First published by Ultimate World Publishing 2025
Copyright © 2025 Debra Stultz

ISBN

Paperback: 978-1-923583-30-6
Ebook: 978-1-923583-31-3

Cover design: Ultimate World Publishing
Layout and typesetting: Ultimate World Publishing
Editor: Marnae Kelley
Back Cover Picture: Mark Webb Photograpy
Supporting contributor: Tyler Burns, MA, LPC, AADC, NCC

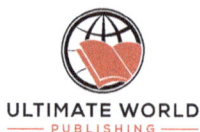

ULTIMATE WORLD
—— PUBLISHING ——

Ultimate World Publishing
Diamond Creek,
Victoria Australia 3089
www.writeabook.com.au

Dedication

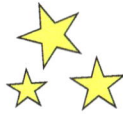

This book is dedicated to my Mother,

Patricia Stultz

whose calm and gentle spirit, unfailing love, wisdom, dedication to our Family, and undying support in all that I do have provided a role model for me to develop a framework of commitment, sincerity, and determination that has contributed to both my personal and professional success.

Mother, I love and appreciate you!

Acknowledgments of Appreciation

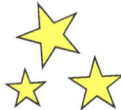

Tyler Burns, MA, LPC, AADC, NCC

I cannot express my gratitude enough to Tyler Burns for his ongoing support and his creative and intellectual contributions to my academic endeavors. Through his editing of my written work, provision of marketing assistance, and offering of design and layout techniques, as well as his artistic input in this book and my other publications, his influence has been priceless. Tyler, I appreciate you very much!

Eugene Aserinsky and the Marshall University School of Medicine

The importance of sleep was relayed to me early in my medical training days, as I had the privilege of having a professor at Marshall

University School of Medicine who was a pioneer in sleep research, Eugene Aserinsky, PhD. In 1953, Dr. Aserinsky helped discover REM sleep. Afterward, with William C. Dement, MD, PhD and Nathaniel Kleitman, PhD, they demonstrated that REM sleep correlated with dreaming and increased brain activity. I also had the privilege of meeting Dr. Dement at a sleep medicine review course at Stanford University. Dr. Dement authored the book *The Promise of Sleep*. Little did I know that they would help to impart such a love of sleep medicine and all things sleep. I am grateful for the opportunity to have been a student of Dr. Aserinsky's and to Marshall University School of Medicine for providing it.

Eugene Aserinsky 1921 – 1998

Mrs. Ruby Dyer, Wayne High School

Few recognize the importance of their high school teachers/sponsors in their day-to-day life as adults. I, on the other hand, totally appreciate the instruction and guidance I received from Mrs. Ruby Dyer at Wayne High School in Wayne, WV. She taught my classes in English, journalism, and yearbook, and was the sponsor for our majorette group. She taught me so much about writing, editing, layout, self-confidence, discipline for achieving your goals, perseverance, standing up for yourself, supervising a team, and being brave. I still use the skills she taught me to this day. I am forever grateful for her guidance!

Testimonials

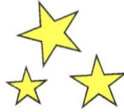

The Power of Restorative Sleep skillfully cuts through the noise of sleep myths and quick fixes to reveal the core truth: better sleep isn't found in chasing unconsciousness, but in understanding what disrupts—and what restores—it. Grounded in science and rich with practical insights, this book reframes how we think about insomnia, sleep apnea, medication, and the many forces that rob us of rest. Whether you're a healthcare provider or someone simply trying to sleep better, this book offers a compassionate and clear evidence-based path forward.

Chris Winter, MD
Author of *The Sleep Solution* and *The Rested Child*
Host of the *Sleep Unplugged* podcast

In this book, Dr. Stultz continues to be a guiding light in the field of sleep medicine! Her ability to blend deep clinical knowledge with heartfelt empathy makes her a rare and invaluable resource for both patients and fellow providers. As a physician in training, I've had the privilege of witnessing her dedication firsthand—whether she's educating patients or families, mentoring students, or advocating for those navigating life with narcolepsy. Dr. Stultz brings clarity to complex conditions and comfort to those who often feel unheard. Her work has a lasting impact on everyone she encounters, and this book is yet another testament to her lifelong commitment to improving patient lives.

Savanna Osburn, D.O., Psychiatry Resident
Marshall University School of Medicine

I have had the privilege of working with Dr. Debbie Stultz for over seventeen years in the field of sleep medicine, specifically in the areas of narcolepsy and Idiopathic Hypersomnia. You will not find a doctor who is more of an advocate for the patients. She treats a variety of different sleep disorders, and there is nothing she won't do to make sure the patients receive the treatment they need and deserve. I would not hesitate to recommend her or this book to any of my friends or family members needing a diagnosis for their sleep disorders. I think it is wonderful that she is now sharing her general knowledge of sleep in this book to help as many patients as possible who suffer from various sleep disorders.

Jimmy Cunningham
Senior Specialty Consultant
Jazz Pharmaceuticals

This book helps to identify many hidden issues that can disrupt sleep and offers practical, easy-to-follow tips for treatment, both for patients and their families. It's not just about getting more hours of sleep, but truly improving the quality of each night's rest, leading to peaceful nights and more energetic, refreshing days.

Asim Roy, M.D.
Medical Director, Ohio Sleep Medicine Institute

Sleep is a fundamental homeostatic process. In order to live, we must sleep. To function optimally, we require adequate quality, quantity, and continuity of sleep. Dr. Debra Stultz not only understands the science of sleep and wakefulness but also possesses a keen insight into the restorative and qualitative aspects of sleep. Dr. Stultz's vast clinical knowledge, research, teaching, and experience have fortunately been effectively shared in this book, *The Power of Restorative Sleep.* Enjoy the read!

Richard Bogan, MD, FCCP, FAASM
Associate Clinical Professor of the University of South
Carolina School of Medicine
Director, Bogan Sleep Consultants
Columbia, South Carolina

Healthy sleep habits are the foundation of every person's well-being. There are many factors that can disrupt healthy sleep, including what you eat, medication, and sleep disorders — the list is long. Dr. Stultz's book provides practical ways to assess and improve your sleep. This is a great read for anyone wanting to learn more about healthy sleep and how to achieve their best night's rest!

Matt Day
Associate Vice President,
HCP Marketing & Head of Remote Sales

Stop the Sleep Stealing!

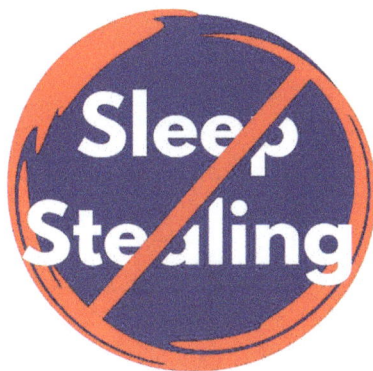

Discover the Ways Within!

Contents

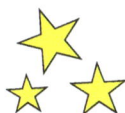

Chapter 1

Introduction and The 3 Ps of Successful Sleep

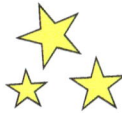

Sleep is a complicated thing!

We all "rob" ourselves of sleep by staying up at night to do one more load of laundry, pay bills, or watch the last episode of our favorite television show. Getting up early in the morning to complete tasks left from the day before, sending an email you forgot to write, stopping for coffee on the way to work, or filling up the gas tank you forgot to fill on your way home the night before can contribute. Sleep is a lot like regularly filling up your car with gas. Without letting your brain and body recharge with sleep, things eventually do not "run" as they should. You may be "sputtering along," but not for long and not without consequences.

Stealing from our sleep in little or big ways, for multiple days per week and several days per month, leads to a "sleep debt" that we can't just repay with one good sleep over the weekend.

The absence of good-quality, deep sleep can lead to many health, mood, cognitive, and relationship issues.

It is well-established that mood disorders lead to disruptions in sleep, but chronic sleep disruptions can lead to depression, mood swings, and irritability. Irregular sleep can undoubtedly make mood swings and bipolar illness more unstable.

Anxiety can increase insomnia and disrupt sleep, and decreased sleep can increase anxiety. Actually, the lack of sleep can be a precipitating event starting a multitude of psychiatric disorders.

In this book, I will focus on the many causes and impacts of insomnia, emphasizing the importance of restful sleep. We will discuss medical disorders that can disrupt sleep, relationship issues, poor sleep hygiene, and taking control of your sleep and daytime alertness. Factors such as sleep schedules, environmental conditions, and lifestyle choices like alcohol and caffeine consumption will be highlighted as contributors to insomnia.

We will examine sleep-conducive environments, including using noise machines, adjusting room temperatures, and avoiding electronic devices before bed.

Behavioral therapies and the importance of the "power hour" routine before sleep will be addressed to help improve sleep quality and overall health.

Key points to be included will be the distinction between REM and non-REM sleep, the role of sleep stages, the importance of allowing sleep cycles to occur naturally, and the effects of disrupted sleep patterns on overall health.

Before we begin, we need to consider the basics of sleep medicine, including how we sleep, and discuss the technical aspects of sleep before tackling more clinical areas. I suggest you take the time to read the first part of the book, as it lays the foundation of knowledge needed to fully understand the consequences of decreased sleep, poor sleep hygiene/routines, and the lack of restorative sleep.

Are You Awake or Alert?

Are you awake or alert each day? The definition of being *awake* is "not asleep."

But are you really *alert* if the only actual requirement to be awake is to cease to sleep? Are you interacting fully with your environment and others if you are just "not asleep"? Being alert implies being fully aware of your surroundings, paying close attention to others and situations of potential danger, and interacting as needed. You need to be alert to drive, interact with your family and coworkers, be productive at work or school, and enjoy the many fascinating aspects of life. Being alert is necessary for safety reasons.

Anything that disrupts or limits sleep can cause you to "go through the motions" of life but not be fully engaged with your environment or others. Our goal in examining the various sleep stealers in this book is to promote awareness, engagement, alertness, improved relationships, increased productivity, and enhanced participation in life that you might otherwise miss out on. Getting enough sleep, getting the right kind of sleep, waking refreshed, feeling energized, and overall wellness can be achieved when you prioritize your sleep, prepare for sleep, and promote healthy sleep. The goal is to be alert, not just awake each day!

Sleep Studies

Let's talk for a minute about how we study sleep. When you first come into our office, you tell us a "subjective" report about your

3

perceived sleep and sleepiness. For instance, what you think the problem is, how much you are sleeping, how you feel the next day, and how your lack of sleep impairs your daily functioning. This gives us a starting point for our evaluation. For example:

- "I am so very sleepy."
- "I only get five to six hours of sleep."
- "My husband's snoring wakes me up all night."
- "I can't function during the day because I can't sleep at night."
- "I never feel rested."
- "I wake up and feel I haven't been to sleep at all."
- "My brain is busy all night."
- "At night, I can't sleep. In the morning, I can't wake up."

Keeping a sleep diary can provide valuable information about your sleep routines and the amount of sleep you are getting and point us in the direction of other issues we may need to address. We often need to do a more "objective" study on your sleep using various forms of in-lab or even a home sleep study. Let me explain some of our testing options:

Sleep diaries/journals are logs you keep at home, including the time you go to bed, how long it took you to get to sleep, what time you woke up, how many times you woke up during the night, what might have contributed to these awakenings, medications or the use of sleep aids, caffeine, or alcohol use, the number and length of any naps you may take, and how sleepy you might feel each day. Tracking this information over several weeks can help identify things that can be suggested to improve sleep quantity and sleep quality. It can also help us determine if additional sleep testing is necessary. Usually, a sleep diary is kept for two weeks. It should be completed daily and not filled out for the whole two weeks at one time, as the daily input is more reliable and provides helpful information. It may be used with actigraphy, as described below.

4

A home sleep test (HST) is a sleep study you do at home after receiving the equipment from your provider's office. It checks your breathing, oxygen levels, and breathing effort and is more for evaluating whether or not apnea is present. It does include oxygen saturation levels and heart rate. It is an abbreviated form of the in-lab study but without as much detail. It does not evaluate for other sleep disorders, such as kicking during your sleep, REM sleep behavior disorder, restless legs, etc.

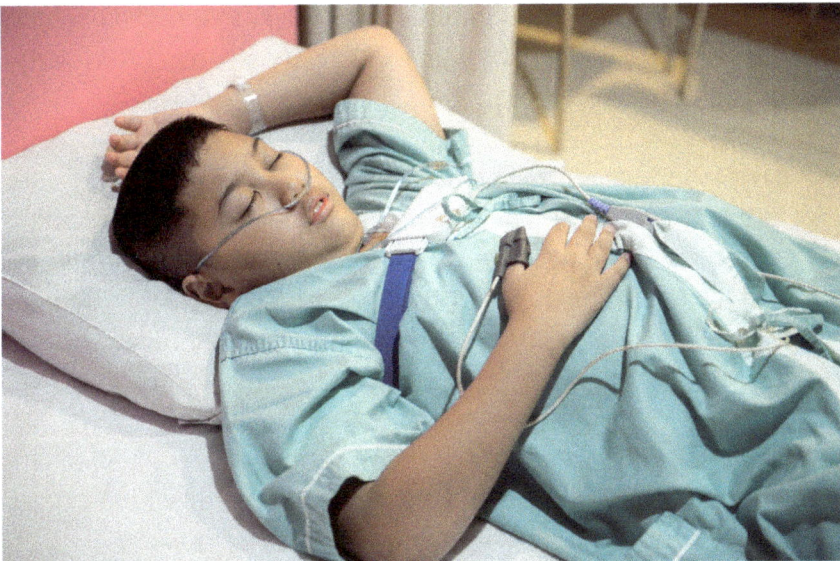

Polysomnography (PSG) is an overnight sleep study in a sleep lab. You are connected to sensors that measure your brain waves, eye movements, heart rate, breathing rate, oxygen levels, leg movements, body position, and whether or not you are snoring. With the PSG, we can stage your sleep and tell whether you are getting all the necessary stages of sleep and enough REM, as well as the deeper, more restorative stage 3 NREM sleep. We can evaluate sleep apnea, kicking during sleep, and restless legs. A cardiac monitor will check the heart rate and for any arrhythmias that may be present.

Sometimes, a PSG must be combined with another type of sleep test, the multiple sleep latency test (MSLT), to evaluate excessive daytime sleepiness.

Multiple sleep latency test (MSLT) is a sleep study done after an overnight PSG study in the sleep lab, in which we look at your degree of sleepiness and the type of sleep you are having. This test helps us distinguish between narcolepsy and Idiopathic Hypersomnia and whether or not substantial sleepiness was documented. It measures how quickly you fall asleep and what kind of sleep you get. The presence of multiple episodes of REM sleep helps to clarify the diagnosis of narcolepsy.

Many prescriptions and over-the-counter medications can interfere with this test. If you are scheduled to have an MSLT, you must share a list of *all* the prescribed and over-the-counter medications you are taking with your sleep specialist, as some will need to be held for up to two weeks or longer before your study. If not, your study may be falsely negative.

Marijuana use is another substance that can interfere with the MSLT findings and needs to be stopped two to three weeks before the sleep study, or else it could negate your test results.

Actigraphy is a sleep monitor worn on your non-dominant wrist or sometimes the ankle to help monitor movement and rest cycles. It can be worn for multiple days to collect data. Actigraphy can provide information on how much you move during the day and night, your total sleep time, sleep onset, wakefulness after sleep, awakenings, and sleep efficiency. It is used in combination with the information from a sleep diary.

The Importance of Sleep

Sleep is part of the foundation of our physical and mental health, as are diet, exercise, social support/interactions, sunshine, etc. We are well aware that becoming dehydrated may result in needing admission to the hospital for IV fluids. Without food, one may suffer from hypoglycemia and decreased energy for daily activities, unclear thinking, resulting in physical sensations of excessive sweating, feeling faint, lightheadedness, shaking, mental confusion, palpitations, headache, and irritability, requiring interventions.

Sleep deprivation can result in a variety of health issues or symptoms, too. We run the risk of increased coronary events if we routinely sleep less than six hours. Other effects include decreased mood, immune function, memory and concentration, hypertension, and weight issues. With slowed reaction time from being sleepy, we may have increased accidents and even falls. Academic and occupational dysfunction, reduced quality of life, increased relationship issues with partners, children, and coworkers, as well as decreased pain tolerance, are more of the consequences of reduced sleep. In addition, some people will self-medicate, creating a cycle of substance misuse or abuse.

Many things contribute to disrupted sleep, including insomnia and other "sleep stealers," which result in lighter, fragmented, or decreased sleep. This book will discuss many potential factors that may lead to unrefreshing sleep. First, let's start with a general overview of insomnia.

Types of Insomnia

The definition of insomnia can include many things, for example:

- Initial insomnia with trouble getting to sleep
- Frequent awakenings throughout the night, or sleep maintenance insomnia
- Early morning awakenings
- Unrefreshing/non-restorative sleep
- Decreased sleep efficiency (the percentage of time spent sleeping while in bed)

Insomnia is also defined by the length of the disorder, such as:

- Acute
- Chronic
- Intermittent

Insomnia is the most common sleep disorder and must cause impairment or distress to be classified as a disorder. Sleep efficiency values greater than or equal to 80-85% are usually considered normal, and less than that would suggest sleep disruption. Sleep efficiency is calculated by dividing your total sleep time by your total time in bed.

Sleep efficiency = total sleep time

divided by the

total time in bed

Risk factors for insomnia include:

- female gender
- advancing age
- lower socio-economic status
- being unemployed
- being divorced or widowed
- shift workers
- poor health status
- medical, neurologic, and psychiatric disorders

"Let her sleep, for when she wakes,
she will shake the world."

~ Napoleon Bonaparte

Understanding Sleep Stages

There's a lot we know about sleep and a lot that's yet unknown. You have sleep stages and sleep cycles. We classify sleep in two categories:

- REM sleep
- Non-REM sleep

REM sleep stands for "rapid eye movement" sleep, the sleep stage in which we do most of our dreaming. During REM sleep, your brain is very active, and your body is paralyzed. The brain waves during REM look very similar to wake brain waves. During REM sleep, your heart rate, breathing rate, and blood pressure increase. We think REM sleep is essential for mood and memory consolidation.

NREM stands for non-REM sleep and is basically everything outside REM sleep.

Non-Rem sleep is further broken down into three stages:

- Stage 1
- Stage 2
- Stage 3

During NREM sleep, your breathing rate, body temperature, and heart rate decrease. Stage 1 is a lighter sleep, barely under wakefulness. Stage 2 is where we spend the majority of our sleep. Stage 3 sleep is sometimes called "delta" or "slow wave sleep." Stage 3 is a deeper, more restorative stage of sleep physically.

During sleep, you usually have more non-REM Stage 3 sleep earlier in the night and more REM sleep later in the night. Anything that causes disruptions in your sleep pattern can lead to increased amounts of lighter, more fragmented, less refreshing sleep. When you have multiple issues causing sleep disruptions throughout the night, you may find a significantly altered total amount of sleep and significantly lighter sleep with frequent arousals or even brief awakenings. Each time you arouse, you restart the sleep cycle, preventing the accumulating total delta slow wave stage 3 NREM sleep.

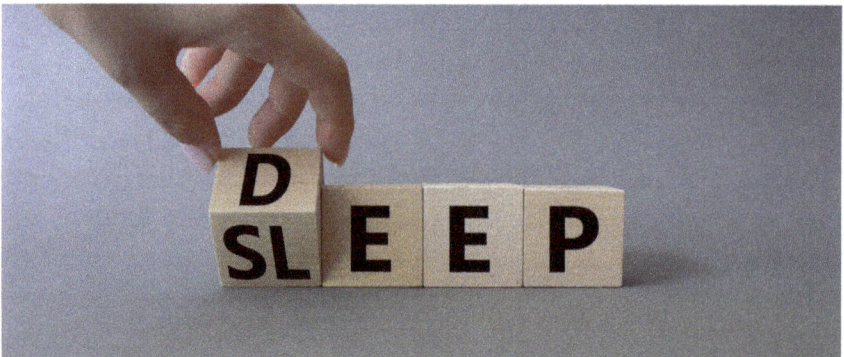

Some patients' sleep is so disrupted by a multitude of issues that they do not have any stage 3 NREM sleep at all. The absence of slow-wave sleep can cause increased pain perception and complaints of excessive fatigue and sleepiness, as well as memory impairment, an increased risk of type 2 diabetes or heart disease, and cognitive decline. These issues will be discussed in further detail in Chapter 11.

At times, it is possible to have what is called "REM rebound," in which your body is trying to compensate for lost REM sleep. It can occur if you have been excessively sleep-deprived, when you first start CPAP, with alcohol use, and even with increased stress. During REM rebound, you may have nightmares, very vivid dreams, increased headaches or migraines, and wake feeling disoriented due to the increased REM sleep. REM rebound can also occur if you are discontinuing medications or situations known to suppress REM sleep, such as various antidepressants, THC, benzodiazepines, or alcohol use.

REM sleep can also be disrupted when someone has narcolepsy, which is associated with excessive daytime sleepiness, irresistible urges to sleep, disrupted sleep, sleep onset REM periods, cataplexy (muscle weakness due to a strong emotion), hypnogogic hallucinations (abnormal visual, auditory, tactile, or kinetic sensations as you are going to sleep) and sleep paralysis (a temporary inability to move or speak while going to sleep or waking). This disorder will be discussed in further detail elsewhere. It is due to the abnormality of REM sleep and timing of sleep, as well as a flickering of sleep during wakefulness and flickering of wake during sleep. It, too, is associated with vivid dreams and nightmares.

In summary, we need enough sleep, each of the different stages and kinds of sleep, the deeper stages of sleep, and uninterrupted sleep for successful acute and chronic functioning. So, it is essential not only *if* you sleep but also *how* you sleep and *how much* sleep you may have at night that is *not interrupted.*

> *"It was that sort of sleep in which you wake every hour and think to yourself that you have not been sleeping at all; you can remember dreams like reflections, daytime thinking slightly warped."*
>
> ~ Kim Stanley Robinson

Causes of Sleep Disruption

Various causes of sleep disruption may have become so common that they are rarely even identified as an issue in patients' complaints of fatigue, insomnia, and non-restorative sleep.

Psychiatric disorders can cause sleep disruption. These include depression, anxiety, OCD, bipolar disorder, PTSD, schizophrenia, panic disorder, and past issues of abuse.

Medical disorders associated with insomnia and nocturnal sleep disruptions include asthma, COPD, thyroid disorders, cardiovascular disorders, nocturnal gastroesophageal reflux disease (GERD), environmental allergies and nasal congestion, renal failure, and chronic pain, to name a few.

Medications such as prescriptions or over-the-counter medications, vitamins, and supplements may contribute to disrupted nocturnal sleep. Examples include decongestants, steroids, inhalers, cardiovascular medicines, statin meds, antidepressants, benzodiazepines, stimulants, nicotine patches, diet pills, birth control pills, antipsychotics, seizure meds, cold/cough medications, diuretics, Parkinson's meds, blood pressure meds, and the list goes on. Please see Chapter 10 for a more complete list.

Neurological disorders associated with insomnia include Parkinson's, dementia, cerebral vascular accidents or strokes, and even head injuries.

Hormonal issues contribute to sleep disruption, such as those occurring during PMS, menopause, pregnancy, decreased testosterone, thyroid abnormalities, polycystic ovarian syndrome, and endometriosis. Hot flashes are also a significant source of sleep issues and frustration for some.

Certain hormones are released during sleep and specific sleep stages. A decreased amount of that stage of sleep can lead to a decrease in hormones, which may cause a particular syndrome or symptoms. For instance, disruption of sleep from sleep apnea can decrease testosterone levels, leading to sexual dysfunction with a decrease in libido and inability to maintain an erection, insomnia, depression, fatigue, reduced ability to concentrate, and increased body fat. Sleep apnea increases the risk of metabolic and endocrine disorders due to the hormonal imbalance from the lack of non-fragmented sleep afforded by regular sleep cycles.

Sleep-related hormones include thyroid hormones, prolactin, testosterone, insulin, ghrelin, cortisol, growth hormone, ACTH, and melatonin. Estrogen and progesterone fluctuations with pregnancy, menopause, and endometriosis can all influence sleep.

Hot flashes are well known to disrupt sleep and lead to increased periods of wakefulness and lighter stages of sleep, more sleep stage changes, decreased sleep efficiency, decreased slow-wave sleep, and a prolonged onset to REM sleep. They can lead to anxiety, palpitations, conflict with sleep partners, and frustration over lack of sleep, all of which can result in irritability and mood issues. Possible treatments for hot flashes will be discussed later in this book.

Substance abuse issues can contribute to sleep problems or creep in as an attempt to self-medicate existing sleep issues. Examples include alcohol use, nicotine use, excessive caffeine use, and even herbal or over-the-counter medications. Alcohol can cause increased nightmares and vivid dreams, as well as restless legs syndrome, increased snoring, worsening of obstructive sleep apnea, increased bathroom trips at night, and even bedwetting. Withdrawal symptoms from any of the above can contribute to disrupted nocturnal sleep and lead to anxiety and restlessness.

Sleep disorders, such as restless legs syndrome, periodic limb movement disorder, obstructive sleep apnea, central sleep apnea, nocturnal leg cramps, nightmares, frequent bathroom trips during the night, and decreased slow-wave sleep, can contribute to disrupted nocturnal sleep.

Other issues associated with sleep disruption include environmental issues, relationship issues, family stress, work stress, having a newborn, young children, and even adolescents newly driving and finding their independence, and chronic pain issues. A history of trauma or sexual abuse is another cause of significant sleep disruption in many.

Sleep trackers and sleep = orthosomnia. Jahrami (Jahrami et al., 2024) reported that orthosomnia is "an unhealthy preoccupation with achieving perfect sleep as defined by tracking devices."

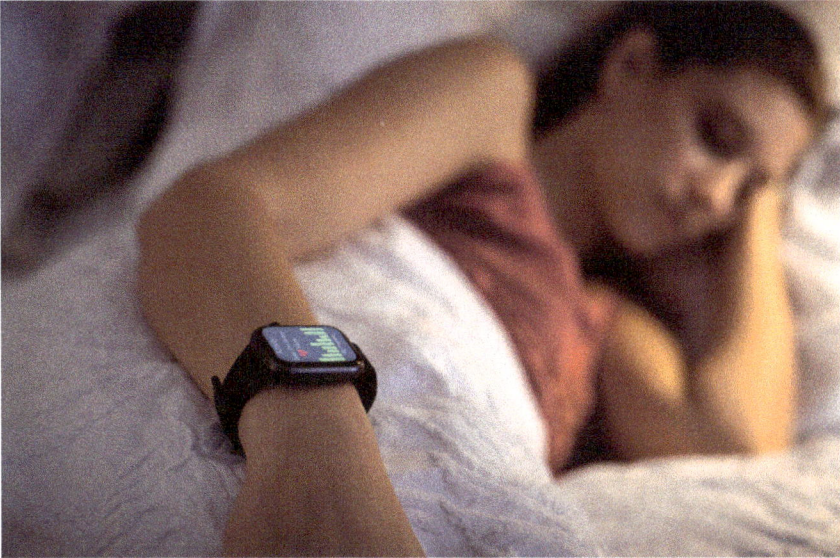

KG Baron et al. coined this term (Baron et al., 2017) in an article entitled "Orthosomnia: Are some patients taking the quantified self too far?" With the growing popularity of sleep trackers on watches, phones, and even beds that have daily sleep tracking reports, users are waking up and predicting the outcome of their day based on the sleep report they obtained from tracking devices.

While much of this book focuses on issues that may be disrupting sleep and causing arousal to lighter stages of sleep, hyper-focusing on sleep trackers can be an obsessive trait contributing to both daytime and nighttime anxiety. Combined with the obsessive search for the perfect pillow, mattress, sleep mask, temperature, etc., you can see why these sleep trackers can lead to obsessive worrying and more disruption than good in some people.

The point of this is to alert you that disturbed nocturnal sleep, insomnia, and feeling unrefreshed the next day may result from many different things clashing together to disrupt sleep significantly. In their totality, this may significantly impact your daily functioning and your physical and mental well-being. We must be aware and look for multiple contributing factors to promote powerful, refreshing sleep!

"It is a common experience that a problem difficult at night is resolved in the morning after the committee of sleep has worked on it."

~ John Steinbeck

As we review the many things that could be contributing to your sleep disruption, I suggest you take notes or highlight areas of concern to return to. Multiple issues usually contribute to insomnia, non-restorative sleep, and excessive daytime sleepiness for the majority of patients who come to my office for evaluation.

What most people want is a little *"fast food"* treatment for their sleep:

"I'll take a little Ambien with a side of melatonin and a large, caffeinated coffee to go, please!"

Instead of taking the time to plan the "menu" for successful sleep by choosing healthy options all day long, they want a quick fix without considering contributing factors, identifying healthy alternatives, and implementing a game plan for consistent restorative sleep.

Sleep disruption requires regulating sleep quantity and quality by examining daytime, evening, and nighttime activities. That is why it is not always a quick fix—not "Here's your Ambien; see you later!"

In our office, we always start our process by having patients complete a comprehensive questionnaire before they are even seen to identify any issues we need to address or investigate further and develop treatment interventions to improve their sleep and daytime functioning. Instead of focusing on one complaint, we look at the bigger picture and tackle as many disruptive issues as possible. To help you, I have included our intake at the back of this book. Please review it, note your contributing issues, and discuss them with your provider.

In this book, I will describe various possible issues that may disrupt your sleep and possible behavioral or pharmacological treatment recommendations. I will not have time to explain an exhaustive list of all the pharmacological treatments, but I will help point you in a direction to discuss with your provider. The field of sleep medicine is growing so quickly that even by the time this book is printed, there will be new options available.

While in scientific writing we usually use generic names for all medications, to aid in familiarity, I will list the most commonly prescribed brand name of the medication, followed by the generic name in parentheses to assist in your understanding.

You may need a provider specializing in sleep disorders if your symptoms are severe. If your provider is unaware of these principles, get them a copy of this book and share it with them, or search for one who does.

The addition of several things contributing to sleep disruption can, in their totality, lead to significant impairment and non-restorative sleep. Addressing as many issues as possible can help dramatically improve your sleep duration and quality. Some of these issues have been so long-standing that it is easy to forget they may be disrupting sleep, or you may have even been unaware that they could disturb sleep.

When you focus only on insomnia or one issue as it contributes to sleep symptoms, you may be prolonging the process of getting to wellness by excluding other possibilities and taking the focus away from other important contributing factors.

After discussing the multitude of things that can go wrong with sleep, I am going to teach you the following:

"The 3 Ps of Successful Sleep"

- **Prioritize your sleep**
- **Prepare for bedtime/sleep**
- **Promote healthy sleep with behaviors all day long**

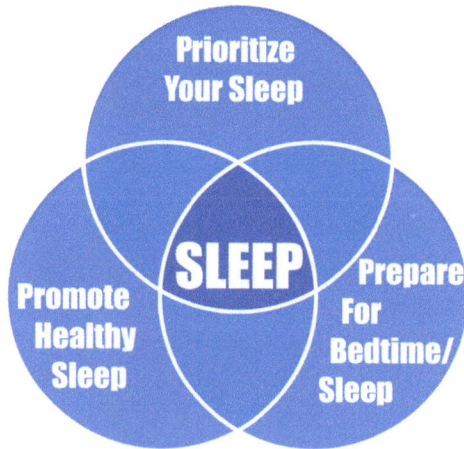

This combo will help your journey to more peaceful nights and energizing days! So, let's begin.

"Sleeping is not time-wasting."

~ Mike Wilson

Chapter 2

If You Sleep Matters!

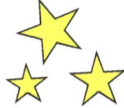

"Sleep deprivation is an illegal torture method outlawed by the Geneva Convention and International Courts, but most of us do it to ourselves."

~ *Ryan Hurd,* Dream Like a Boss: Sleep Better, Dream More, and Wake Up to What Matters Most

One of the first issues to consider is whether or not you prioritize sleep and plan enough time in your day to have a healthy amount of sleep at night. Whether your behaviors during the day and evening time help to promote sleep, like sun exposure, exercise, avoiding caffeine after 3–4 PM, limiting alcohol in the evening, prioritizing your mental health, having healthy, supportive relationships, allowing for "down time" in the evening before bedtime, considering environmental issues that may make sleep less inviting and restorative, limiting electronics for at least an hour before bedtime, reviewing the medications you take at night, etc.

Too often, we are all "running on empty" when it comes to sleep, rest, healthy eating, and stress. If we run our car with little gas, low oil, low tire pressure, an uncharged battery, without routine check-ups, etc., it will break down sooner or later. The same is true for our bodies, which need physical and mental rest and recharging at night with sleep.

Some people can run ok getting 6–7 hours of sleep, but most need 7–8 hours. What happens when you have prolonged nights of only 5–6 hours? How long can you sustain that? Not very long is the answer. If we are chronically sleep deprived, we are building a "**sleep debt**" that influences mood, concentration, memory, anxiety, and frustration tolerance, makes you more distractable, increases your chances of accidents, contributes to relationship issues, contributes to academic and occupational problems, contributes to weight gain, decreases immunity, and increases the risk of medical diseases such as high blood pressure, strokes, heart disease, and diabetes. (Yes, I did say that... not sleeping enough can cause you to gain weight!)

So, just like a bank account where you repeatedly withdraw without the funds to pay, consistently stealing from your sleep each night can create a "sleep debt" that will be hard to overcome. Eventually, your body takes over, and the consequences can be severe.

Take time to review your routine sleep schedule and determine your sleep needs! Prioritize allowing enough time for sleep and rest each day.

"I finally got eight hours of sleep.
It took me three days, but whatever."

~ Unknown

Sleeping too much or too little makes a difference. Some sleepy people sleep up to 10–14 hours, and you know what they say about "too much of a good thing"! Having to sleep that much is disruptive, too! We'll review Hypersomnia and prolonged sleep in Chapter 12 on sleep disorders, discussing narcolepsy and Idiopathic Hypersomnia.

Age-Related Sleep Issues

I will give a brief explanation of a few age-related presentations of illnesses associated with sleep disorders here, including Alzheimer's and Parkinson's in the elderly, pregnancy and sleep, and commonly found sleep disorders in children. Chapter 11 will describe the other sleep disorders in more detail. Most of the issues discussed in this book apply to adults, children, and the elderly, although they may present slightly differently in the different age groups.

Children

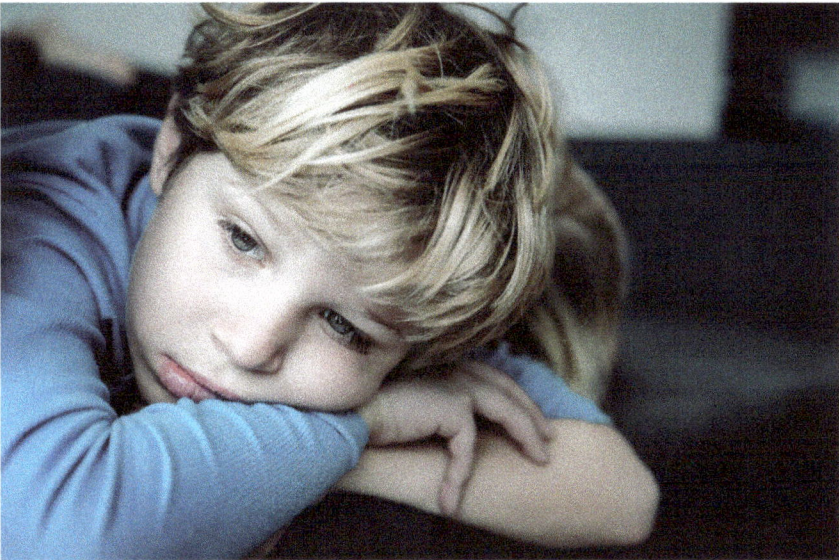

I think we often ignore sleep issues in children and downplay their complaints of insomnia and excessive sleepiness. Usually, their sleepiness presents itself as irritability and is attributed to oppositional actions and behavior disorders. Sleep issues frequently found in children include restless legs syndrome, snoring, disrupted sleep due to sleeping with pets in the room, anxiety, depression, fear, and nightmares or night terrors. Sleepwalking, teeth grinding (bruxism), poor sleep hygiene or chaotic sleep routines, hunger, bed wetting (enuresis), and insomnia may occur.

Insomnia in children can be related to fear, separation anxiety issues, and the desire for increased time with their parents. It can be transient, conditioned, or behavioral. Restless legs syndrome is a relatively common cause of insomnia in children, causing an excessive desire to move, stretch, or scratch the legs. It is usually related to iron deficiency in children, and a multivitamin with iron may be helpful. RLS in children is often dismissed as "growing pains."

We must remember that children get depressed and anxious, too, which can contribute to difficulty getting to or staying asleep.

Sleep apnea and snoring in children are usually related to enlarged tonsils; therefore, a tonsillectomy may be curative. Sinus, allergy issues, and increased weight may also contribute to snoring, loud breathing, and upper airway resistance in the pediatric population, leading to fragmented sleep or excessive daytime sleepiness.

Night terrors are an NREM sleep phenomenon where the child suddenly awakens scared, panicked, and even yelling without remembering what happened. They may be kicking, confused, inconsolable, crying, and thrashing about. These, of course, are very scary and disruptive to the other family members. The child often goes back to sleep with little to no memory of the event, even when questioned the next day. Night terrors are frequently associated with a fever, prior sleep deprivation, certain medications, increased caffeine, or when sleeping in a new place. Other sleep disorders, such as sleep apnea or reflux, or increased stress may precipitate them. Night terrors can run in families.

Nightmares are usually less intense and occur during REM sleep, and the child may remember the dream's content in great detail.

Narcolepsy is a disorder of excessive daytime sleepiness and often starts in childhood with "sleep attacks," where the child suddenly falls asleep or sleeps excessively. Cataplexy (muscle weakness or collapse with strong emotions like laughter or anger) may occur, as can sleep paralysis (where they wake up and briefly feel they cannot move), excessive napping, and sometimes even hyperactivity can occur in children with sleepiness. Cataplexy in children may be associated with slurred speech, jaw weakness, a protruding tongue almost looking "Downs-like," and facial movements looking almost like tics. Or it can occur with arm, hand, or leg weakness. These episodes may be triggered by laughter (or when preparing to tell a joke), anger, fear, excitement, or any strong emotion. Patients with narcolepsy can have fragmented sleep and insomnia, as well as "brain fog" and difficulty concentrating. Narcolepsy in children is often associated with sudden weight gain and the early onset of puberty. Sleepiness may be misattributed to mono, laziness, depression, thyroid disorders, etc.

Narcolepsy in children may have symptoms similar to ADHD, especially if cataplexy is not present or recognized. The diagnosis of narcolepsy is often missed for many years, even though early symptoms may be present in childhood.

ADHD and Sleep

ADHD has long been associated with sleep disorders such as insomnia, restless legs syndrome, poor sleep hygiene, poor sleep quality, delayed circadian rhythms, snoring, nightmares, and even sleep apnea. Daytime sleepiness, trouble with concentration/ memory, irritability, or mood issues may be due to ADHD, sleep disorder symptoms, or medications to treat ADHD. A careful assessment is advised, including a detailed sleep history, a sleep diary, and information from parents and teachers. In my opinion, screening for sleep disorders should be a routine part of any evaluation for the treatment of children or adolescents with ADHD. Treatment of sleep apnea may improve symptoms thought to be ADHD. Pediatric narcolepsy can present with symptoms similar to ADHD and result in the misdiagnosis of narcolepsy for many years.

Delayed sleep onset, circadian rhythm disorders, excessive caffeine use, sleep deprivation, and substance abuse can be associated with ADHD or present with symptoms like ADHD in the adolescent population. Clinical history is essential with adolescents in the evaluation of ADHD symptoms, as well as a urine drug screen.

Sleep architecture changes may be demonstrated in both pediatric and adolescent ADHD symptoms. Lunsford-Avery et al. (2025) studied sleep in adolescents with and without ADHD. They found increased sleep disturbances, lower amounts of stage 3 NREM slow wave sleep, increased amounts of stage 2 sleep, and more complaints about sleep, which were associated with lower cognitive performance in those with ADHD. Demonstrating again it is not just if you sleep but how you sleep that may contribute to dysfunction.

Adolescent and College-age

Adolescence and young adulthood may be characterized by an obsession with electronics and gaming, which may dominate activity and impair sleep. Chapter 9 will discuss electronics and sleep. Electronics cannot be overlooked as a cause of sleep disruption in this population, and often, parents, significant others, and providers may not even realize how late they are staying up and disrupting their sleep. A careful history can help determine their sleep schedule, caffeine use, blue light exposure, and nighttime stimulation from games with friends that may contribute to poor performance, decreased grades, decreased social involvement, excessive sleepiness, safety concerns, etc.

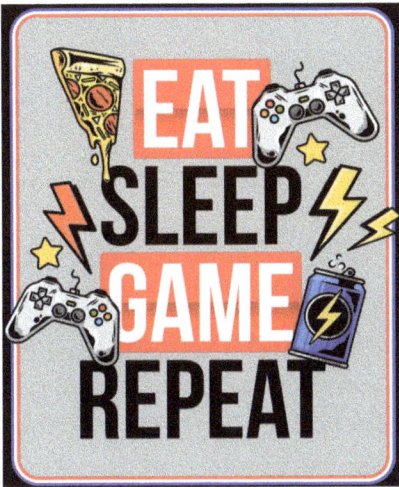

Adults

Many sleep disorders are common in the adult population and will be covered in Chapter 11. At this point, I would like to highlight sleep issues associated with pregnancy, breast cancer, and hot flashes.

Pregnancy and Sleep

An article on the Sleep Foundation website entitled "Pregnancy & Sleep: Common Issues & Tips for Sleeping" by Danielle Pacheco and reviewed by Ealena Callender from March 27, 2024, outlined the importance of sleep during pregnancy for both the Mother and the Baby. They reported that poor sleep is related to gestational diabetes, developing high blood pressure during pregnancy, preeclampsia, immunity issues, and possibly preterm birth, low birth weight, depression, cesarean delivery, and painful labor. They also suggested there is emerging evidence that poor sleep may contribute to sleep problems and crying in babies once they are born. The article indicated obstructive sleep apnea may occur in as many as one in every five pregnancies, and restless legs syndrome can occur in a third of women in their third trimester.

Causes of sleep disruption during pregnancy:

- Snoring or even sleep apnea can occur with weight gain and nasal congestion due to hormonal changes
- Pressure, physical discomfort, or pain
- Inability to get comfortable
- Frequent bathroom trips
- GERD (gastroesophageal reflux)
- Restless legs syndrome
- Leg cramps
- Breast tenderness
- Back pain
- Round ligament pain during the second trimester, which occurs in the abdomen, hips, or groin area during pregnancy
- Insomnia in the past with exacerbation during pregnancy
- Anxiety about the future, worrying about the delivery process, worrying about the baby, relationship concerns
- Hormonal changes
- Morning sickness and nausea
- Shortness of breath from hormonal changes and the growing baby taking up room
- Contractions
- Having a very active fetus with lots of movements at night
- Postpartum depression

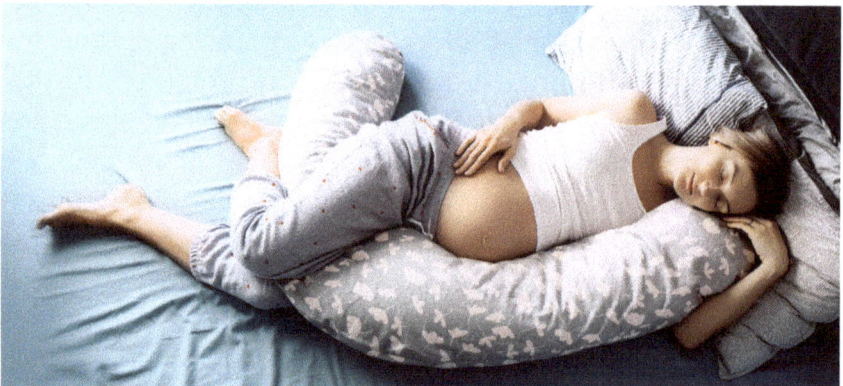

Advice for sleep during pregnancy:

- Use a pregnancy pillow.
- Keep to a routine day and night.
- Elevate the head of the bed or use a wedge pillow to decrease reflux.
- Avoid eating, drinking excessive fluids, or caffeine in the afternoon or evening to prevent bathroom trips and promote sleep.
- Avoid late afternoon or evening naps.
- Sleep on the left side with the legs slightly curled.
- Avoid sleeping on the back to prevent backaches and putting pressure on the vena cava, which can cause dizziness and prevent good blood flow to the baby.
- Follow general insomnia guidelines listed in Chapters 12 and 13 of this book.
- If anxiety or depression are prominent, seek therapy or medication intervention.
- Establish a bedtime routine and be aware of your sleeping environment.

Breast Cancer and Sleep

Getting the diagnosis of breast cancer is traumatic to the system and often especially sleep. Daldoul (Daldoul et al., 2023) studied seventy-nine patients with breast cancer and found 40% had clinically significant insomnia, 13% had clinically significant depression, and 21% had clinically significant anxiety. Insomnia was significantly associated with depressive symptoms, anxiety symptoms, and fatigue. Patients with clinical insomnia had a lower ability to function physically, less ability to function in general, less energy, more bodily pain, more problems with mental health, and a lower ability to function socially. Hot flashes were reported by 68% of patients with clinically significant insomnia.

Disrupted sleep in breast cancer can be due to:

- Hot flashes
- Pain
- Depression
- Pre-existing sleep disturbances
- Psychological distress
- Nocturia
- Other sleep disorders—obstructive sleep apnea, restless legs, periodic limb movement disorder
- Relationship issues
- Self-esteem/body image issues
- Increased alcohol use
- Chemotherapy or medications to treat breast cancer

Night Sweats/Hot Flashes

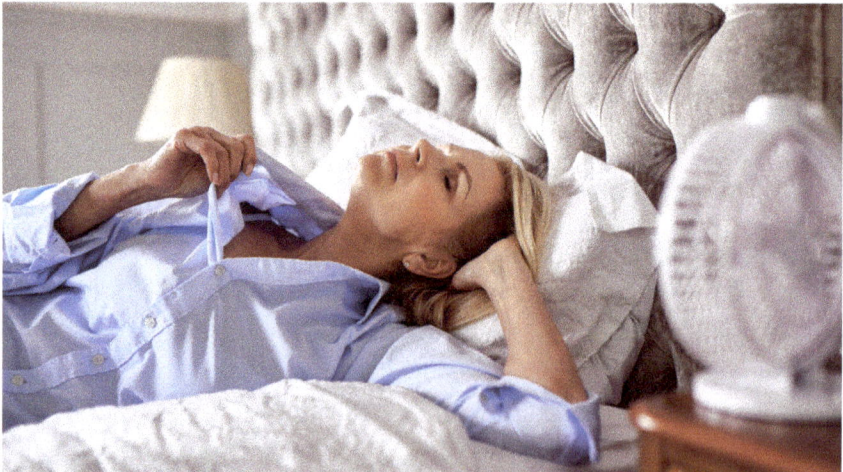

Hot flashes and sweating commonly occur during the perimenopausal and menopausal periods in females. They can also occur during pregnancy. Other causes of night sweats include medications such as chemotherapy, antidepressants, antihypertensive drugs, methadone, steroids, medications to treat endometriosis, or birth control pills. Anxiety and stress may increase nocturnal sweating by increasing the release of hormones that cause sweating. Environmental issues such as too many covers, a hot room, bed partners, and pets sleeping too close can cause nocturnal sweating. Metabolic issues such as hyperthyroidism, diabetes, and hypoglycemia, as well as infections such as mononucleosis, Lyme disease, endocarditis, HIV, and tuberculosis, can cause night sweats. Certain cancers, such as breast cancer, prostate cancer, lymphoma, and leukemia, have also been associated with nocturnal sweating. Alcohol use or substance abuse and autoimmune disorders are other causes. Sleep disorders such as obstructive sleep apnea can cause nocturnal sweating. Spicy foods or hot drinks before bedtime can be an issue, too. Vitamin B12 deficiency can cause spinal cord abnormalities, leading to autonomic sympathetic hyperactivity and drenching night sweats. Iron deficiency can also cause night sweats. Dehydration can cause night sweats, and excessive night sweats can lead to dehydration. Hyperhidrosis is a condition that involves excessive sweating day or night for no apparent reason, and Glycopyrrolate is often used for its treatment and can be taken at night.

So, the first treatment for night sweats is identifying and treating all contributing issues.

Treatments that have been used for night sweats or hot flashes include:

- Vitamin E
- Magnesium
- Fish oil
- Wearing breathable clothing
- Avoiding hot and spicy foods before bedtime

- Avoiding dehydration
- Megestrol acetate
- Clonidine
- Hormonal therapy with estrogen with or without progestin if hot flashes are menopausal-related
- Certain SSRI antidepressants, such as Effexor (venlafaxine) or Paxil (paroxetine), are often used. Brisdelle is a form of paroxetine that is FDA-approved to treat hot flashes and contains only 7.5 mg of paroxetine.
- Veozh (fezolinetant) is a non-hormonal treatment for menopausal hot flashes.
- Neurontin (gabapentin) or Lyrica (pregabalin)
- Combo of Effexor (venlafaxine) and Ambien (zolpidem)
- St. John's wort
- Black cohosh
- MENO vitamins for menopause that include black cohosh and ashwagandha
- Oxybutynin
- Trazodone
- Vitamin B12 and/or B6
- CBT (cognitive behavioral therapy)
- Use gel pillows or mattress covers developed for cooling.
- Place a cold pack under your pillow and flip it as needed to create a cool sleeping surface.

Elderly

Two common diseases in the elderly are very often associated with sleep disorders and will be discussed here, including Alzheimer's and Parkinson's. Restless legs syndrome is also widespread in the elderly due to anemia, multiple medications, and coexisting health disorders and will be discussed in detail in Chapter 11.

Alzheimer's

Alzheimer's is often associated with abnormal sleep schedules with frequent napping, and studies have demonstrated that not getting enough sleep can be harmful and even lead to dementia.

Wennberg et al. wrote an article entitled "Sleep Disturbance, Cognitive Decline, and Dementia: A Review" (Wennberg et al., 2017) discussing this topic, reporting 60–70% of people with cognitive impairment or dementia have sleep disturbances, which are linked to poorer disease prognosis. The article focused on both Alzheimer's and Parkinson's, as well as the treatment of insomnia, daytime sleepiness, sleep-disordered breathing, and REM Behavior Disorder. They concluded that since sleep is a modifiable behavior, its treatment has the "potential to determine the trajectories of dementia, improve prognosis, and reduce the risk of poor clinical outcomes in these disorders." They summarized that "sleep disruption, sleep duration, and sleep disorders—specifically SDB (sleep disordered breathing)—all may increase the risk of all-cause cognitive decline and dementia. Conversely, populations with clinical levels of cognitive decline, including AD (Alzheimer's Disease), exhibit elevated sleep disturbances. A bidirectional link appears to exist between sleep and dementia."

Andrew E. Budson, MD, wrote an online article at www.health.harvard.edu entitled "Sleep well—and reduce your risk of dementia and death" (2021). In it, he outlined two different studies discussing the risk of decreased sleep and the development of dementia and other health issues.

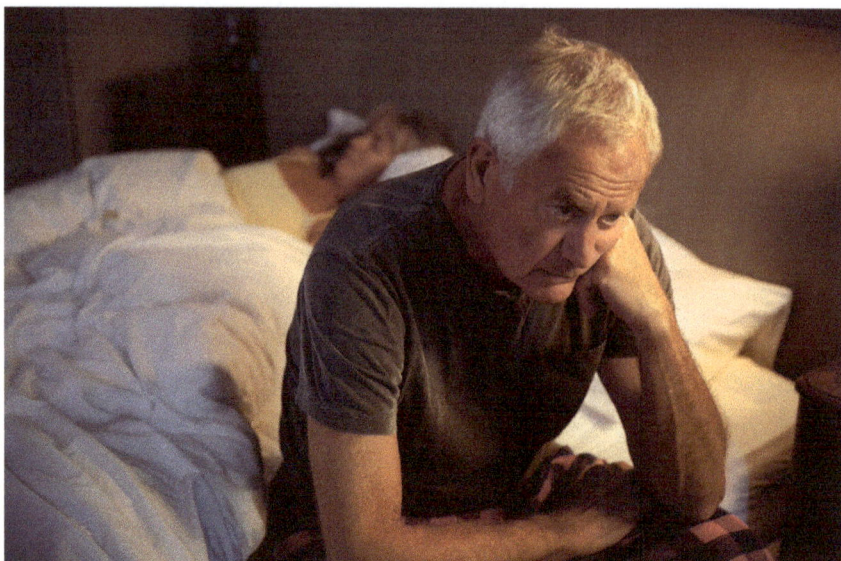

A study from Harvard Medical School by Robbins et al. entitled "Examining sleep deficiency and disturbance and their risk for incident dementia and all-cause mortality in older adults across 5 years in the United States" (2021) studied 2,800 people ages 65 and older and found that individuals sleeping less than 5 hours per night were twice as likely to develop dementia and twice as likely to die compared to those sleeping six to eight hours per night.

The second study in their article discussed 8000 participants in Europe and found that consistently sleeping less than 6 hours at ages 50, 60, and 70 years old was associated with a 30% increased risk of developing dementia.

These studies demonstrate the risk of not sleeping and dementia. Once patients develop Alzheimer's, they can be sleepy during the day, not sleep at night, and have more confusion at night.

Up to 25% of those with mild or moderate dementia have sleep issues, and 50% of those with severe dementia have sleep issues. Sleep issues with Alzheimer's include trouble getting to sleep, waking too early, feeling sleepy during the daytime, frequent napping, increased confusion as the afternoon or evening arrives called "sundowning," sedation from medications, depression, anxiety, grief, and coexisting health issues causing sleepiness such as sleep apnea and restless legs syndrome. Just because they have Alzheimer's, we should not dismiss the impact of other mental, physical, or environmental issues as causing sleep problems and contributing to their confusion.

The following are some suggestions for helping dementia patients with sleep issues:

- Limit naps and dozing during the daytime, especially later in the day, to help promote sleep at night.
- Keep them busy with activities during the day and early afternoon.
- Give them their baths or have them take showers earlier in the day to avoid overstimulation at night.
- Slow down the activities and stimulation in the evening to encourage sleep at night.
- Remember, chronic pain, sleep apnea, restless legs syndrome, nocturia, reflux, and all the other sleep disruptions described in this book can still be an issue for them at night and need to be addressed aggressively. Treating these disorders can help the patients and their caretakers sleep better.
- Use music from "their time" to relax and improve their mood in the evening.
- Focus on their strengths and abilities—not just disabilities!
- Have them be productive and complete simple activities for as long as possible to maintain their cognitive stimulation and self-esteem.
- Don't try to correct, reason with, or confront them, especially in the evening, as that can increase frustration and escalate anxiety issues before bedtime.

- As dementia advances, they may spend a lot of time sleeping but do not forget about coexisting depression as a cause of increased sleep. Treating depression may help make symptoms more tolerable for everyone.
- Also, consider they may just be bored. Audiobooks, old movies or television shows, chair exercises, word search books, coloring, listening to music every night around 7 PM, and often providing some routine to their schedule may help.
- Light therapy and exposure to daylight earlier in the day may be helpful.
- Look at the medications they are on that may be contributing to insomnia, excessive daytime sleepiness, or increased bathroom trips at night. Even medications causing constipation and abdominal pain can be disruptive. Making sure they go to the bathroom to empty their bladder just before bed should be one of the last things they do at night before bedtime.
- Don't dismiss their chronic pain issues and aggressively try the behavioral interventions discussed in Chapter 8 of this book for pain.
- Consider melatonin.
- Consider aromatherapy, such as lavender, on their wrists or temples at nighttime.
- If indicated, consider a multivitamin with iron to help with nutritional deficiencies caused by eating less. This may also help decrease restless leg symptoms.

Parkinson's Disease

Parkinson's is a neurodegenerative disease found in the elderly associated with sleep disruptions such as insomnia, excessive daytime sleepiness, restless legs syndrome, sleep apnea, and another sleep disorder called REM behavior disorder (RBD). This disorder will be covered further in Chapter 11. Still, briefly, it is a disorder of REM sleep in which the normal paralysis of REM sleep is "unhooked," and patients are allowed to act out their dreams physically. It can sometimes lead to vocalizations or yelling out, physical movements or aggression, singing, and even harm to their bed partners or themselves. RBD occurs in about 25–50% of patients with Parkinson's. RBD can occur with other disorders and situations, too, such as dementia with Lewy Bodies and multiple system atrophy. It can precede the diagnosis of Parkinson's by many years.

Many other age-related issues may exist in the pediatric and geriatric populations and during pregnancy. These issues must be identified and addressed to promote restorative sleep and mental and physical wellness.

Chapter 3

When You Sleep Matters!

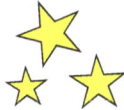

It is not just *if* you sleep; it is *how much* you sleep and *when* you sleep.

Having a disrupted sleep-wake schedule matters!

A circadian rhythm is your body's natural clock, which usually runs over a 24-hour cycle and is influenced by light and dark cycles. However, it can also be influenced by various things, such as physical activity, food intake, sleep habits, temperatures, brain injuries, neurological disorders, travel between time zones, and sunlight exposure.

Circadian rhythm disorder is sleeping outside a normal 24-hour circadian sleep rhythm. Those who go to sleep too early and wake too early have an advanced sleep phase type, and those who go to sleep too late and wake too late have a delayed sleep phase type and are often called "night owls."

Circadian rhythm disorders include shift work sleep disorder, delayed sleep phase syndrome, advanced sleep phase syndrome, non-24-hour sleep-wake rhythm disorder, jet lag, and irregular sleep-wake rhythm disorder.

Shift Work Sleep Disorder

"With 10 million Americans wrestling with shift work, their internal clocks are like puzzle pieces out of place."

~ Matt Walker @sleepdiplomat

Professor of Neuroscience and Psychology at the University of California, Berkeley

One of the clearest examples of "when you sleep matters" is demonstrated in those working shift work. Shift work can vary so much that the brain (and the body) never knows if they are coming or going. Disrupting the circadian system by sleeping at different times and decreasing total sleep can be extremely frustrating and confusing. Often, they can't sleep on demand when they have time to rest and can't stay awake when they must. Overall, they are usually functioning in a chronic sleep-deprived state associated with cognitive issues, possibly mood/anxiety disorders, slower reaction times, irritability, or gastrointestinal symptoms.

"Shift work makes 8-hour sleep a dream—It's a square peg in a round hole for your 24-hour rhythm due to circadian misalignment."

~ Matt Walker @sleepdiplomat

Shift work refers to any schedule outside a person's regular routine. To some, working from 7 AM to 3 PM is difficult because they may have to get up by 5–6 AM to make it to work on time. Some people are well-adjusted to the evening shift because they are used to staying up late and sleeping in. Usually, the overnight shift is an issue for anyone because they stay up during the day running errands, picking up kids, going to their children's sporting events, having meals with the family, going to doctors' appointments, and then rush to get a few hours of sleep before they have to get to work at 11 PM...and then they stay up all night and have to stay alert enough to drive home before repeating the cycle.

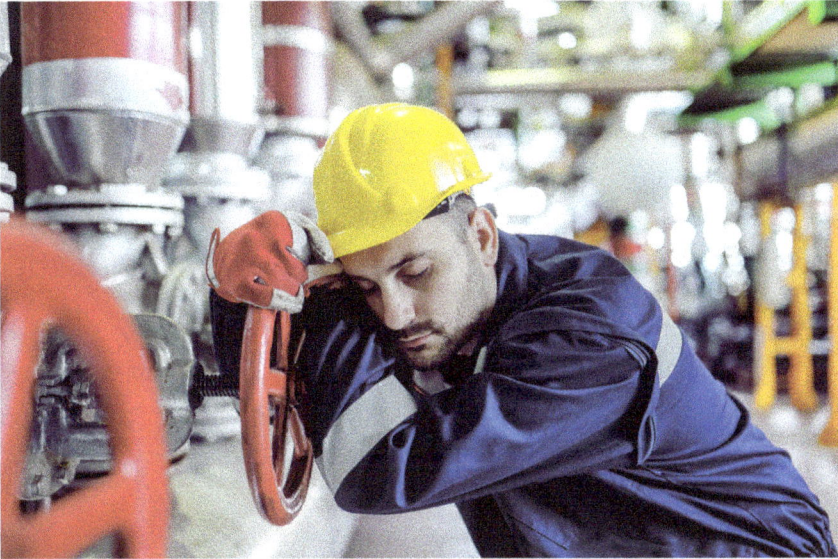

Shift work is associated with trouble getting to sleep, staying asleep, waking up, and feeling sleepy and unrefreshed during working hours.

Shift work has been associated with an increased risk of obesity, high blood pressure, gastrointestinal issues, headaches, mental health disorders/depression, low frustration tolerance, diabetes, breast cancer, decreased testosterone levels, poor work performance, increased clumsiness, and accidents, including motor vehicle accidents.

"It took just three years of working extreme night shifts to wreck my health."

~ *Steven Magee,* Night Shift Recovery

Anyone working shift work should be aware of safety issues when driving after being awake for extended periods. Substance abuse may also become an issue in some as shift workers may self-medicate with alcohol, stimulants, or other drugs to both stay awake and go to sleep.

Sometimes, when symptoms are excessive, people who work shifts may need a prescription sleep aid for their "night" and a "wake-promoting" medication during their working hours. Wake-promoting medications such as Nuvigil (armodafinil) and Provigil (modafinil) are FDA-approved for shift work sleep disorder. We will discuss these medications in a later chapter.

Tips for surviving shift work include the following:

- Rotating shifts in a forward direction (towards a later work schedule)
- Limiting the number of consecutive shift workdays (less than three when possible)
- Limiting overtime work
- Limiting commute times to and from work
- Avoiding alcohol
- Protecting the bedroom with dark shades, room-darkening shades, or even cardboard or aluminum foil placed in the windows to prevent the sun from coming in and disrupting sleep
- Using sound machines to muffle environmental noise
- Overlapping of sleep schedules by 30% on days off

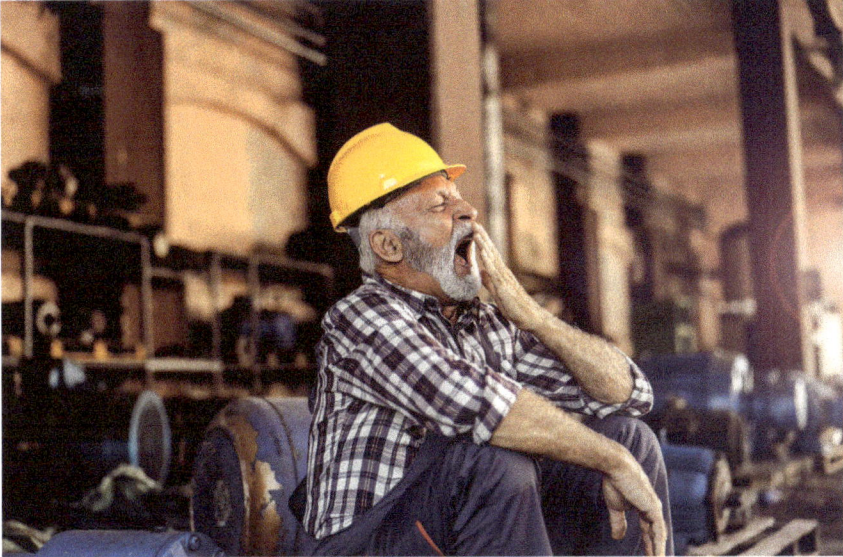

- Dark sunglasses or welding glasses when leaving work during the daytime to limit sun exposure and enhance the ability to sleep when arriving home
- Sleep masks to limit light exposure (some even have the ability to play music or white noise to decrease sleep disruptions)
- Practicing good sleep hygiene (this will be discussed more in chapters 12 and 13)
- Taking naps right before evening or night shift work
- Light therapy before work may promote alertness. Light therapy boxes, such as those used for seasonal affective disorder, can be purchased online and must be **10,000 lux** in intensity.
- Every attempt should be made to limit disruptions from family members, the phone, the doorbell, etc., during sleep to allow periods of uninterrupted sleep and progression of all sleep stages. Place "Do not disturb" or "Please be quiet" signs on the front door, around the doorbell, and the bedroom door.

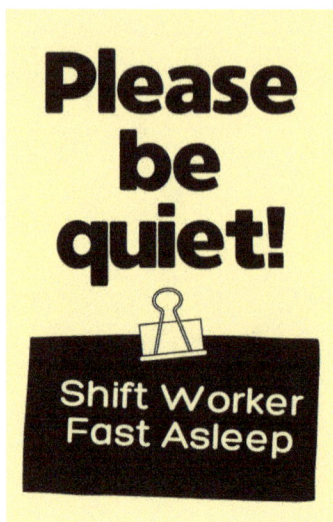

Please be quiet!

Shift Worker Fast Asleep

Plan doctor's appointments and other activities at a time that is least disruptive to sleeping schedules.

"I would run down like a battery during my extreme night shifts, and I would never fully recover during the week off between them. I would start my next set of extreme night shifts in a sickly state."

~ Steven Magee,
Night Shift Recovery

Delayed Sleep Phase Syndrome (DSPS)

Delayed sleep phase syndrome is a circadian rhythm disorder in which people go to sleep very late and sleep late. It is common in adolescents, which makes it very difficult to get up for school in the morning and be alert. It is also common among "gamers" who stay up late playing video games with friends late into the night. It is usually defined as going to sleep at least two hours later than the standard desired sleep times.

Delayed sleep phase syndrome can cause academic, occupational, and relationship problems. It is often associated with daytime sleepiness, impaired memory/concentration, and complaints from friends or family members. It often runs in families and patients with this disorder may do better working evening or midnight shifts and not scheduling early morning appointments.

*"I think sleeping was my problem in school.
If school had started at four in the afternoon,
I'd be a college graduate today."*

~ George Foreman

Treatment recommendations for DSPS include the following:

- Light therapy can be beneficial in increasing light exposure in the early morning hours between 6 and 9 AM.
- Decrease light exposure in the evening.
- Avoid caffeine after 6 PM.
- Avoid exercising two to three hours before bedtime.
- Melatonin may be helpful, but the actual dose and timing of treatment are unclear. It is suggested that melatonin be taken in the early evening for DSPS, and it has been used with light and/or chronotherapy.
- Sedatives often have minimal benefit for this disorder except when taken at higher doses.
- Chronotherapy is a behavioral therapy that delays sleep by two to three hours every two days until the desired sleep time is achieved. Then, the schedule must be maintained, and weekend "sleep-ins" should be avoided.
- Avoid bright computer screens and gaming after 11 PM. Also, turning down the brightness of the computer even earlier, at 9–10 PM, can help, and/or using gaming glasses in the evening. These glasses can be ordered online and are blue-light-blocking for computers, TV, and gaming use, which can decrease eyestrain and reportedly promote melatonin production. Remember, melatonin is a hormone that helps regulate sleep, and blue light slows melatonin production.

Advanced Sleep Phase Syndrome

Advanced sleep phase syndrome (ASPS) is a circadian rhythm disorder in which people go to sleep much earlier and wake up earlier than desired. Their internal clock is off. They are likely to go to sleep between 6 and 9 PM and wake between 2 and 5 AM. They get enough sleep, but it is at the wrong time. ASPS is often seen in the elderly and can run in families. It is also associated with autism spectrum disorder. Their focus on early morning awakenings and feeling as if they are not getting enough sleep can be disturbing.

This disorder can also be treated with bright lights, but the timing of the light exposure is different. It is usually used in the evening, 1–2 hours before bedtime. The goal is delaying sleep by 20–30 minutes each night until a more appropriate bedtime is achieved. Melatonin may also help readjust the sleep schedule and can be given at bedtime or halfway through the night.

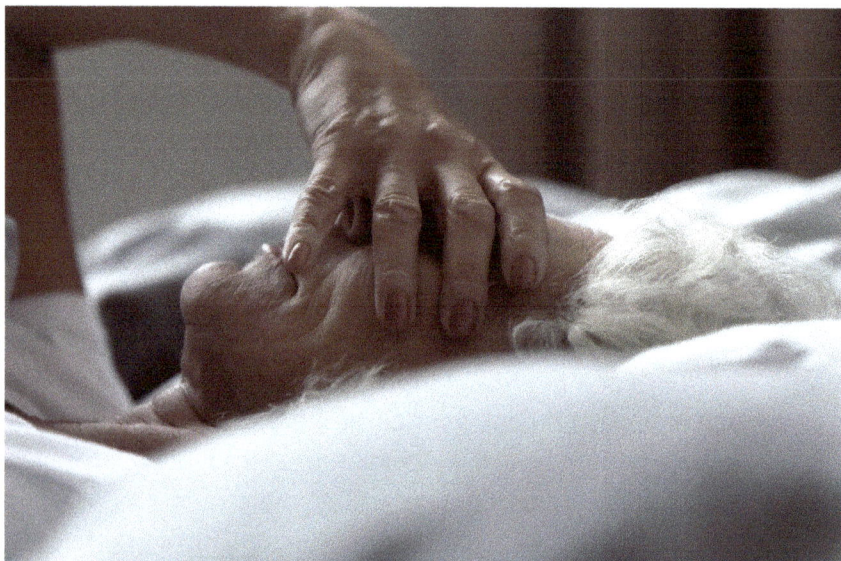

A sweet little lady I treated with this disorder came to me with complaints of insomnia, stating she woke every morning between 4 and 5 AM. Initially, we were focused on ruling out obstructive sleep apnea as she snored. She also had some restless leg symptoms that we treated. She repeatedly told me she fell asleep just after the news and woke "in the middle of the night." After an extensive workup, including labs and a sleep study, she was diagnosed with and treated for primary snoring and restless legs syndrome. She had continued complaints. After reviewing the history again to see what we may have missed, I learned that she was going to bed each night after *the 6 PM news*, not the 11 PM news! She was in bed from about 7–7:30 PM each night and up by 4–5 AM. She was getting more than enough sleep, but the focus was on the early morning awakenings and insomnia complaints. Lesson learned: Always ask which news show they are talking about!

But this brings up many interesting points. The definition of insomnia can be different for everyone. Multiple issues may contribute to unsatisfying sleep, and the history...the whole history...the specific history...is essential. We must always look for the possibility of more than one issue contributing to the symptoms.

This is one reason I have patients complete such an exhaustive questionnaire before being treated. There may be multiple issues, including depression or psychiatric problems, contributing to insomnia, multiple medications confusing the picture, and various symptoms the patients don't even connect as being relevant. A sleep diary can also be important, especially if completed correctly.

Non-24-Hour Sleep Wake Disorder

Non-24-hour is a circadian rhythm disorder most commonly seen in patients who are blind and lack the typical light-dark exposure needed to set their sleep rhythm. It can also occur in those who are not blind. It is also seen after head injuries, brain tumors, dementia, and autism. It is more commonly seen in young males.

With this disorder, the internal sleep schedule is off to the point that the patient goes to bed later and later, wakes up later each day, and fails to synchronize to a 24-hour day. It can be longer or shorter than 24 hours. Body temperature and hormone rhythms are also off. Their sleep is not aligned with the typical 24-hour day, causing social, occupational, and educational difficulties. Sleep can be delayed so much that it eventually cycles back to a standard sleep time before being disrupted again. It is very confusing and frustrating for the patient and loved ones.

Hetlioz (tasimelton) is an FDA-approved treatment for non-24-hour sleep disorder. It is a melatonin receptor agonist. Light therapy, chronotherapy, sleep hygiene, exercise, cognitive behavioral therapy, supportive therapy, and psychoeducation are also helpful interventions for the patient and their family.

Irregular Sleep-wake Rhythm Disorder

Irregular sleep-wake rhythm disorder is a rare circadian rhythm disorder in which patients have no clear sleep/wake pattern. Their sleep occurs in random on-and-off naps with no explicit sleep episodes. This disorder is associated with disrupted sleep, increased daytime sleepiness, and abnormal total sleep time. It occurs more in the elderly but can occur in children with neurodevelopmental disorders such as autism and other developmental disorders. It can be seen with mental health disorders, brain injuries, Parkinson's disease, Huntington's disease, and dementia, and in those not exposed to enough light.

Sleep usually occurs in short intervals throughout the day with no particular routine, which can be difficult for the patient and their family members or caretakers.

Treatment is similar to the previously mentioned disorders, such as using bright light therapy, melatonin, sleep hygiene, structured daily activities/mealtimes, and behavioral therapy.

Jet Lag

When people travel across two or more time zones, their routine body rhythms can be out of sync with the daytime and nighttime demands of the new time zone, causing jet lag symptoms of sleepiness, trouble sleeping at the time delegated by the new time zone, gastrointestinal issues, difficulty concentrating and functioning during the new "wake" schedules, causing irritability and mood problems. The body's internal clock is out of rhythm with the world's external clock's demands. The more time zones away from the routine schedule, the more difficulty one may have. Flying east is harder than going west. How long you will stay in the new time zone will determine how much you need to try to adjust your sleep. If you will only be there for one or two days, staying on your usual time zone schedule as much as possible is advisable. If your stay is extended, you must adjust to accommodate.

Tips to aid with jet lag include:

- Adjust your sleep/wake schedule to the new schedule for a few days before your trip.

- Avoid being sleep-deprived before you travel.
- Melatonin may be helpful.
- Drink plenty of fluids as you travel and stay hydrated.
- Light therapy may be helpful. For example, if traveling west, expose yourself to light in the evening; if traveling east, use light therapy in the morning.
- Napping to recharge may make adjusting more tolerable, but don't make naps too long.

Excessive Napping

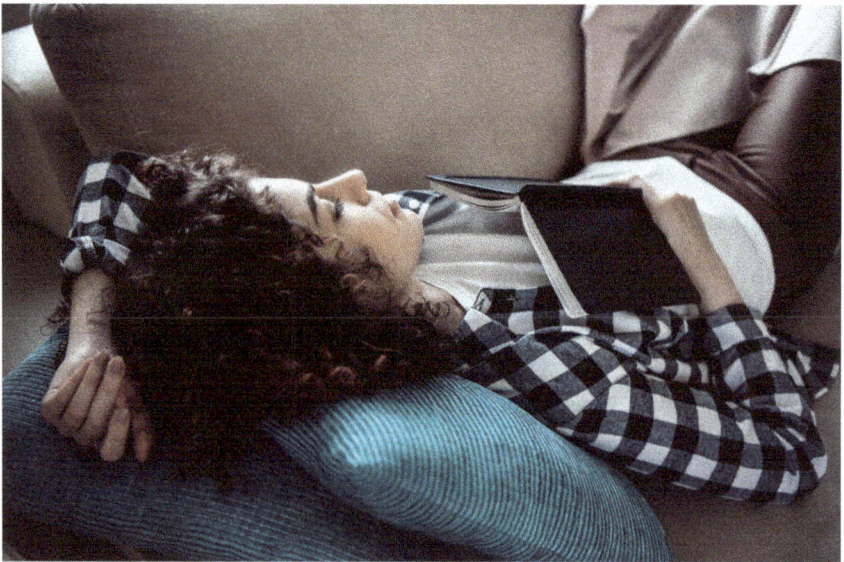

Various issues can cause excessive napping and disrupt the sleep-wake schedule, leading to prolonged disruptive sleep patterns. Increased napping may be seen with depression, dementia, grief, boredom, medications, substance abuse, bipolar disorder, seasonal affective disorder, head injuries, and other sleep disorders such as narcolepsy and Idiopathic Hypersomnia. In narcolepsy, naps are usually brief (20–30 minutes) and restorative, unlike the long, unrefreshing naps of Idiopathic Hypersomnia. Some people with significant anxiety use naps as a way to avoid things. Medical issues can contribute to frequent napping, such as thyroid disease, chronic fatigue syndrome, mononucleosis, or anemia. With depression, some people nap because they are so discouraged and hopeless.

Taking a multi-hour nap in the afternoon may affect nighttime sleep. If this is a reoccurring pattern, your sleep cycle can become unbalanced, creating instability. Sleeping too long in the afternoon prevents getting enough sleep at night, contributing to daytime sleepiness. This results in long naps after work, and then the cycle repeats.

A sleep diary can help identify this pattern. Treatment of the underlying or associated issue/disorder can improve daytime wakefulness, allow for more consolidated sleep at night, and promote more productive and alert days.

Chapter 4

Where You Sleep Matters!

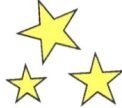

⭐⭐⭐

"Oh bed! Oh bed! Delicious bed: That heaven upon earth to the weary head."

~ Thomas Hood, Author

Your sleeping environment does matter! This would include everything from the temperature of the room to the light in the room, the clutter in the room, the comfort of the mattress, the support of the pillow, having enough covers but not too many, the absence of outside noise, actually sleeping in a bedroom and not on the couch, who else is sleeping in the room, unresolved emotional issues with your bed partner, having pets in the room or children in the room, and the list goes on and on.

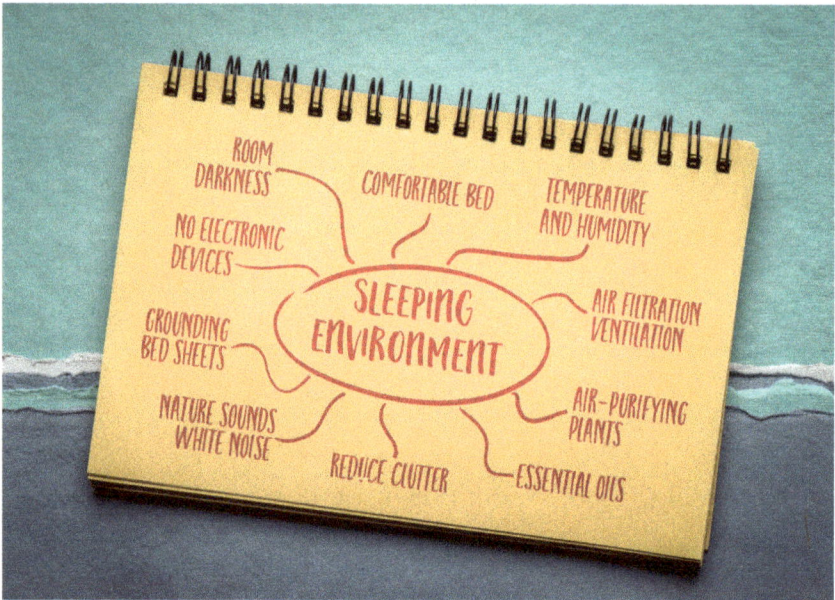

Stepping back and taking a conscious look at your room during the day can help you figure out what you need to do to make your bedroom a sleeping environment that is peaceful, relaxing, free of distractions, comfortable, and the most sleep-promoting it can be. We will have a whole chapter on electronics in your room and another on sleeping with snoring partners, kids, and pets—all of which can disrupt sleep. For now, we will focus on other environmental issues.

As I have said before, your sleep issues and daytime sleepiness may be due to many small things that can snowball, significantly impacting your physical well-being, mental/emotional health, and occupational and educational performance. We need to identify and address as many of these small things as possible because they can lead to significant results for your sleep! Something as simple as getting a new pillow may help you sleep better, have fewer headaches, snore less, have less neck pain/stiffness, and help you to wake more refreshed.

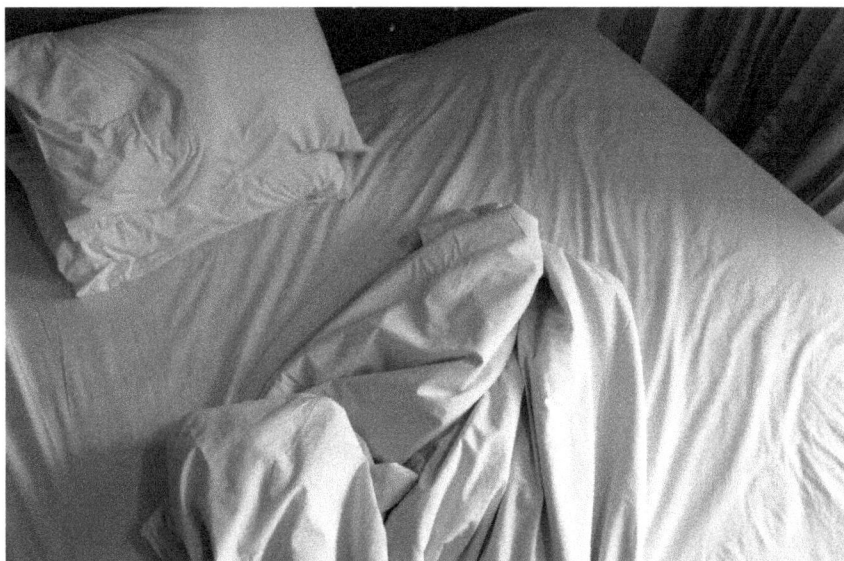

The same can be true for an older mattress that has lost its padding and firmness, developed ruts or imprints of where you sleep each night, or even have springs poking you during sleep. An old mattress can become saggy, contributing to back pain and non-restorative sleep. It can make noise and disrupt your sleep with its creaking, popping noises, or squeaking as you or your bed partner toss and turn. Even if it does not entirely wake you, it can arouse you to a lighter stage of sleep and prevent stage 3 NREM slow-wave restorative sleep.

If you can't afford a new mattress, get a 3–4 inch memory foam mattress topper. They are much more affordable these days. If you can afford a new mattress, do your homework. Investing in sleep and your health can be incredibly beneficial. Upgrading the mattress you use each night can make a big difference.

If you have a bed partner who snores or the two of you like different temperatures or amounts of covers on your bed, invest in split adjustable beds. Raise the head of your snoring spouse's bed. Add an electric blanket to your side of the bed. Whatever you need to do to make your sleep more restorative is what you need to do, and this can cut down on conflict and be relationship-building!

Now, some beds respond to snoring automatically, and there are some with lumbar support, sleep coaching, under-bed lighting, sound machines, head and foot lifts, USB and USB-C ports, massage, and remotes.

One of the women who used to work in our office had a bed that had an "AI Sleep Coach" attached that sent her daily text messages stating such things as:

- "Last night, 20% of your sleep was deep sleep, which is a nice improvement over your average of 12% from the prior 7 days. Your physical health and immune system will reap the benefits of adding deep sleep."

- "Pavlovian sleep trick. Some say you can teach your body to know when it's time to fall asleep. Pick a habit, such as rubbing the tip of your nose, pulling an earlobe, or squeezing your upper arm, and do it each night before you fall asleep. The idea is that your body will eventually accept this motion as a signal that it is time for it to rest."

These beds are like having your own personal sleep coach cheering you on each night! Another few of her bed's tips were:

- "Monkey around. If you are still hungry after dinner, bananas make a good snack: they are great natural sources of the sleep hormone melatonin and the sleep-inducing tryptophan."

- "Makes scents. Try this essential oil recipe for sound sleep: 15 drops lavender, 10 drops vetiver, 5 drops each of frankincense, ylang-ylang, and wild orange. Combine in a 10 ml roller bottle and top off with fractionated coconut oil. Apply to feet and neck."

I would be tempted to get this bed just to get the daily text messages! If you are wondering, she has the TEMPUR-ERGO ProSmart® with the Sleeptracker-AI®, but I think several other brands have the same technology. I believe the Sleeptracker-AI® program works with other mattresses, too. This is not a commercial for that mattress brand; I thought you might be curious after telling you the story.

There are also adjustable firmness mattresses where you can adjust for firmness or softness on the different sides of the bed and other "Smart Beds" to choose from. A review of all of these is beyond what I can provide here. One hint I might have for you is if you go away on a trip and have a fantastic night of sleep due to the comfort of the bed, ask the hotel what type of mattress they have or what pillows they use. You can look at the Sleep Foundation website for further information.

Sometimes, adjustable beds also help with chronic pain issues. Some beds with "zero gravity" adjust to keep your head, knees, and legs slightly above your heart to make breathing easier. Elevating your feet when there is swelling in your extremities, elevating the head of your bed if you have sleep apnea or snoring, and adjusting for sciatica and back pain can all be beneficial.

If you have issues with gastroesophageal reflux, an adjustable bed or sleeping on a triangle wedge pillow may also help decrease reflux and sleep arousals and lead to deeper, more restorative sleep.

Also, consider the sheets you use. Sleepfoundation.org reviews so many sleep-related items that you may find helpful, including sheets, mattresses, pillows, pajamas, sleep masks, sleep trackers, wake-up lights, alarm clocks, etc.

If your room is dusty, it could contribute to nasal congestion, snoring, upper airway resistance, and non-restorative sleep. Dust often, run the sweeper often, change your sheets and pillowcases often, replace your pillow periodically, and add dustproof covers to your pillows. If you are already on allergy medication, you may want to try taking it at night. Pet dander from pets, dust mites from stuffed animals, and fuzzy bathrobes and blankets may contribute to allergies, nasal congestion, coughing, and even asthma or respiratory issues. Wash stuffed animals in a pillowcase frequently and/or put them in a low dryer for about 20 minutes to remove dust mites to help your children breathe and sleep better. Consider these things if you wake up congested, snoring, or have any allergy symptoms.

Light in and around your room can be disruptive. I know some people who like to sleep with no lights on in the house at all because they find it disruptive. I want a small light in the bathroom to see the way when I get up. Some living in apartments may have a flashing light outside from a neighboring business. Many shift workers may have to sleep during the daytime hours. If light coming through your room is an issue, invest in room-darkening shades or curtains. Another option would be to put cardboard or tape black plastic bags or aluminum foil on your windows to block the light. It sounds extreme, but restorative sleep is necessary.

Sleep masks help block out light and may be purchased online. Some even come with sound, Bluetooth technology, massagers, electric eye heat for dry eyes, unique designs for side sleepers, 3D options, weighted options, or with lavender, etc.

The temperature in your room can make a difference. Some people like a very cool room with many covers, while others like their bedroom to be warm. The problem with a very warm room is that during REM sleep, your body does not regulate temperature well, and being too warm can cause sleep arousal.

The Sleep Foundation (sleepfoundation.org), in a March 2024 article posted on their website by Danielle Pacheco and Dr. David Rosen, reported, "The ideal temperature for sleep is between 65–68 degrees; thermoregulation during sleep is a crucial factor to sleep quality, and your body's temperature naturally drops as you sleep, so a cooler room makes it easier to fall asleep and stay asleep." They added, "this may vary by a few degrees from person to person." I am very cold natured, and my son's room is downstairs, which is much cooler in our house, so I usually keep our thermostat at around 68–70 degrees. So, there is some variability, but generally, being too warm causes more disruptions to sleep, and the Sleep Foundation post states a higher core body temperature has been associated with decreased restorative slow-wave sleep, reduced sleep efficiency, and a higher likelihood of waking. Programmable thermostats can be one way to vary temperature settings at night, promote healthy sleep, and warm things up a little when you have to get up in the morning.

Having excessive clutter in your bedroom can also make a difference. We want your room to be as peaceful and serene as possible. Having multiple books lying on the other half of your bed (I am guilty of this), laundry all over the room, workstations in your bedroom with bills, mail, work articles, etc., does not allow your mind to slow down and your body to relax. A cluttered space can increase stress and cortisol levels. Your body and mind may not associate this room with your resting place, your sleeping quarters, or your place to turn off and tune out the world's chaos.

Do a 10-minute declutter, straighten and turn down your covers for sleep, pick one book or magazine that is more relaxing to read, and dim the lights. I love a good legal murder mystery, but if I start reading it at night, I will stay up late and lose sleep every time. Choose what you read at night carefully.

If you have a TV in your room, try watching a comedy or relaxing show rather than an intense drama, shoot-em-up show, or the news. Listen to soft music, meditate, or pray. Consciously choose every aspect of your sleeping environment to promote the onset and maintenance of sleep. Lavender and other essential oils, such as cedarwood, chamomile, bergamot orange, and ylang-ylang, to name a few, have been reported to be relaxing and aid in sleep. If you have trouble the next day, rosemary and peppermint have been used for alertness, anxiety, and cognitive functioning. Cinnamon has been suggested by some for concentration. There are some fascinating articles on aromatherapy for sleep, alertness, relaxation, brain fog, etc.

Avoid using your bed for anything but sleep and sex. Do not hang out and fret. If you can't sleep, get up, do some non-stimulating activity in another room, and try going to sleep again later. We do not want your bed to be associated with worry and restlessness. Your bed should be a place of relaxation, respected for rest, and not the place for difficult conversations or relationship stress. Plan difficult relationship discussions around 6–8 PM after dinner when you are not exhausted and not in bed. Refrain from conflict right before bedtime. Honor your sleeping space!

Chapter 5

Who You Sleep with Matters!

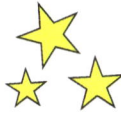

This question often sounds funny when I ask a patient about it, but it matters. Sleeping with a spouse or partner who snores or kicks excessively can be very disruptive. If you sleep with children who move around a lot, kick, tend to sweat, and do not self-soothe well, your sleep may be interrupted every few minutes, leading to lighter stages of sleep, frequent sleep transitions, and non-restorative sleep.

Those cute little pets can also often be a significant issue. I had one patient who got up each night around 3–4 AM and went outside with their dog to take a walk and a bathroom break. No matter the outside temperature, rain, snow, etc., they were up in the middle of the night. She reported she quickly went back to sleep; however, as stated previously, it can disrupt your sleep cycle and your ability to obtain the deeper stages of sleep.

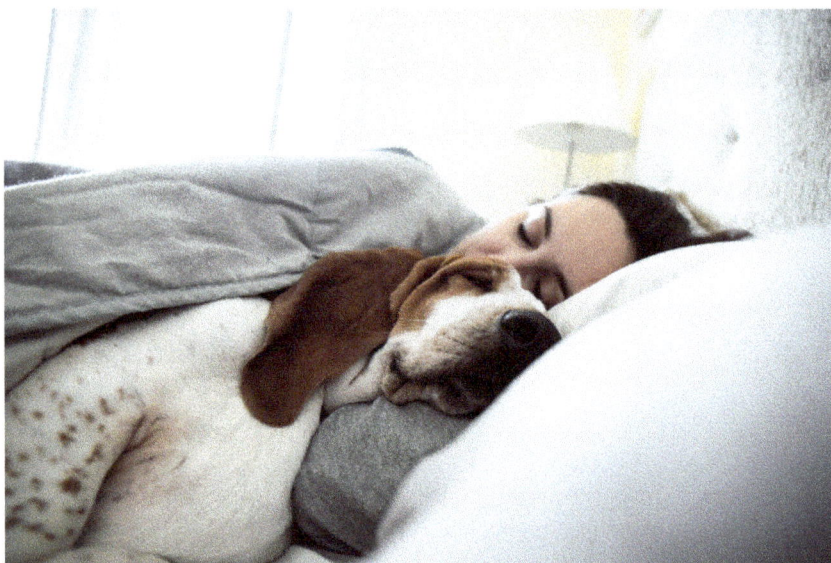

Pets quickly "train us" to be on their schedule. The midnight walks became a habit for the dog, but she still had to work each day and get up early each morning. Getting up in the cold and even in the rain or snow in the middle of the night disrupts routine sleep restoration.

"First, they steal your heart. Then they steal your bed."

~ Unknown

I once treated another patient for insomnia, unrefreshing sleep, and depression who, upon further review of their history, slept with a snoring spouse and two Great Dane dogs! At least they had a king-size bed, but the ability to have deep, restorative, non-disrupted sleep was obviously "greatly" impaired!

Dogs dream during their sleep and may bark out, growl, twitch, kick their legs, or make other noises or movements that can be disruptive to those trying to sleep with them. And obviously, size matters, as two Great Danes would take up a lot of sleeping space.

Cats purring, playing, and deliberately trying to wake you during the night are common issues as they are naturally nocturnal. They may be hungry, thirsty, bored, or lonely. If they wake you and you immediately feed them, they may learn to expect that on a routine basis. If they wake you and then you pet and love on them, they will learn to do that behavior more often. Try ignoring them so as not to reinforce this behavior. It is probably best to have them sleep in another room with the door closed where their bed, food, water, and toys are available and their litter box is clean. Some attention to them before bedtime may help prevent them from demanding attention during the night. If you have issues with sleep or allergies, you should probably not let pets sleep in your bed, as nasal congestion can lead to snoring, possibly increased apnea, and fragmented sleep. You can pay more attention to them and try to love on them twice as much during the waking hours before bedtime.

Hamsters and sleep do not play well together! I once went on a trip and stayed in the bedroom of my friend's children, who had a hamster. I could not believe how disrupted my sleep was! Hamsters are most active from dusk to dawn and sleep in multiple cycles during the day. They tend to run on a hamster wheel most of the night. If you are a light sleeper, that can be torture. Even if you are not a light sleeper, it can disrupt regular sleep cycles for humans, depriving them of deep sleep.

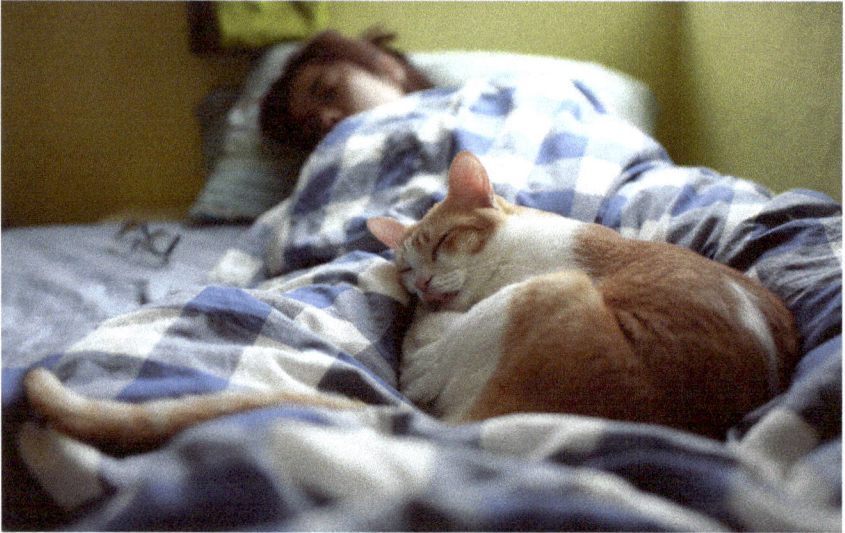

I once had a child referred to me for anxiety and to rule out psychosis from a local pediatrician. When we got down to it, she had four to five animals sleeping in her room, including a hamster. When we gave her a little something for her mood/anxiety and cleared the animals out of her bedroom, she was back to normal in no time. So, remember your children and their need for restorative sleep, too, when you allow pets in their bedroom!

Speaking of children, let's talk about letting your kids sleep in your bed. I was a single Mom, and my son had colic. I let him sleep in my room as a necessity for me to get some sleep early on, which proved to be a hard habit to break. I knew the rules even back then, but I was in survival mode while having to get up early for work.

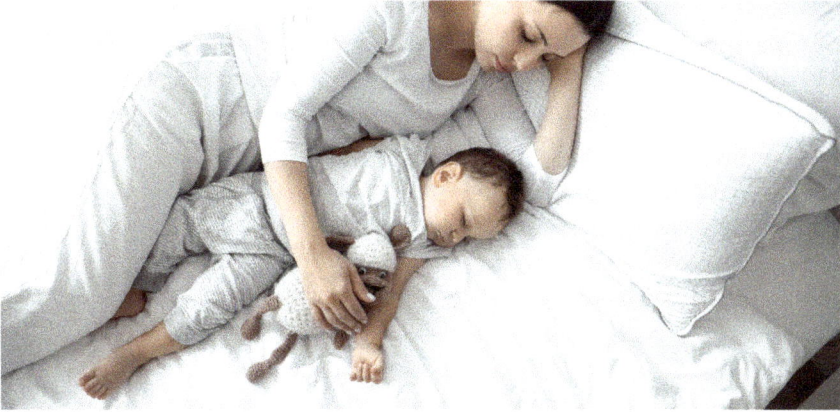

With respect to infants, the American Academy of Pediatrics recommend room sharing without bed sharing for at least six months, with the infant close to the parents' bed. Using a separate area such as a crib, bassinet, moses basket, bedside sleeper, or portable play yard to reduce the risk of sudden unexplained infant death syndrome (SUIDS) is suggested. They recommend placing your baby on its back on a firm, non-inclined, flat sleep surface, while avoiding soft objects, loose bedding, or other things that could increase the risk of danger. In fact, they should be placed on their back for the first year. Keeping your baby warm but not too hot is encouraged by using extra layers of clothing instead of blankets.

As they get older, an occasional sleepover with your kids in your room can be fun, but if they kick, move excessively, snore, or wake up excessively, it can disrupt your sleep. It is also essential for them to learn self-soothing techniques and good sleep habits early on in life.

Now, let's talk about your snoring spouse. We will discuss sleep apnea in Chapter 11. Still, suppose your bed partner is snoring and having pauses in their sleep, gasping, waking unrefreshed, or has coexisting blood pressure, heart, or other health issues. In that case, they need to be evaluated for obstructive sleep apnea. Their life could depend on it, and the potential for developing other health risks could depend on it! Not everyone who snores has sleep apnea, and not everyone with sleep apnea snores. If they are kicking or twitching throughout the night, they could have another sleep disorder. Evaluating them for sleep disorders is not just about your comfort and sleep. It is crucial for their future health.

Another forgotten issue is that the loud snoring can also lead to resentment from the other bed partner, causing relationship stress and even a "sleep divorce" where people sleep in different rooms. More on this later.

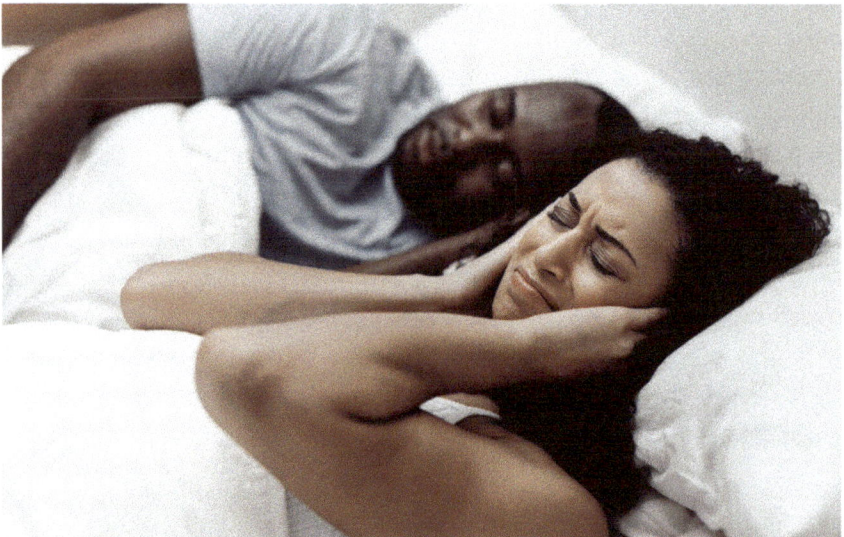

Chapter 6

Mental Health Matters!

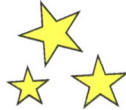

*"The best bridge between despair and
hope is a good night's sleep."*

~ E. Joseph Cossman

There are a variety of mental health issues that can contribute to
or cause issues with sleep. Also, sleep disorders and other things
that disrupt sleep can lead to depression, irritability, mood swings,
anxiety, concentration/memory problems, decreased energy,
and lack of motivation. Both depression and sleep problems are
bidirectional. Depression, bipolar disorder, anxiety disorders, and a
host of other mental disorders can all contribute to sleep disruption.
A brief review of the Diagnostic and Statistical Manual of Mental
Disorders (DSM-5) (American Psychiatric Association, 2013) criteria
for these disorders will be reviewed here. This is not an exhaustive
review of all of the psychiatric disorders, and I would direct you to a
mental health professional if needed for evaluation and treatment
if you are experiencing symptoms suggestive of a mental disorder.

Depression/Dysthymia

By the DSM-5 definition, depression is associated with the following and occurs most days for more than two weeks:

- Decreased mood, feeling sad, feelings of hopelessness, worthlessness, or irritability
- Decreased or increased sleep nearly every day
- Decreased or increased appetite and weight
- Decreased energy or psychomotor agitation
- Decreased concentration or indecisiveness
- Decreased interest or pleasure
- Decreased motivation
- Increased feelings of guilt or worthlessness
- Thoughts of death or suicide

"Sleep is not on good terms with broken hearts. It will have nothing to do with them."

~ Christopher Pike

Depression is further classified as major depressive disorder, occurring for at least **two weeks** duration, or dysthymia (persistent depressive disorder), which is a chronic depressed mood for more days than not over **at least two years** duration. In children, dysthymia can also present as irritability and only needs to be present for at least one year. Dysthymia is also associated with insomnia or hypersomnia, low energy or fatigue, and other symptoms of depression.

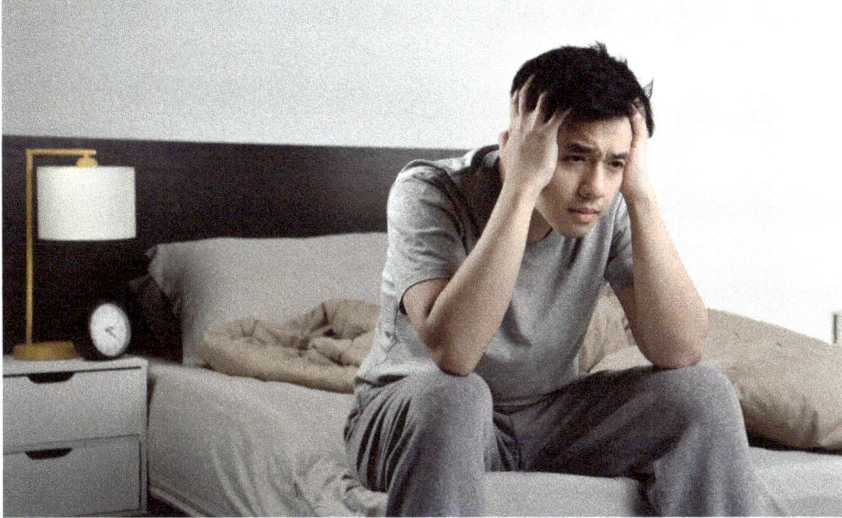

Sometimes, even the treatments for depression can contribute to insomnia and disrupted sleep, such as SSRI antidepressants like Prozac (fluoxetine), Zoloft (sertraline), and Lexapro (escitalopram) or the SNRI antidepressants like Effexor (venlafaxine) or Cymbalta (duloxetine) and meds such as Wellbutrin (bupropion).

Other antidepressants can make you sleepy and are often used to treat insomnia, such as Elavil (amitriptyline), Pamelor (nortriptyline), Silenor (doxepin), Remeron (mirtazapine), or Desyrel (trazodone). We often use sedating antidepressants when both symptoms of insomnia and depression are present and also use sedating antidepressants to treat insomnia even if depression or anxiety are absent.

Some antidepressants, such as Cymbalta (duloxetine) or Effexor (venlafaxine), can increase restless legs syndrome and disrupt sleep. Medications and sleep will be discussed further in Chapter 10.

Mood Swings and Bipolar Disorder

Bipolar disorder is diagnosed when there have been significant mood swings with distinct episodes of manic moods, which are abnormally elevated or irritable moods for at least one week associated with:

- Inflated self-esteem or grandiosity
- Decreased need for sleep
- Increased talking
- A flight of ideas or racing thoughts
- Distractibility
- Increased goal-directed activity
- Excessive impulsive involvement in activities such as sexual indiscretions, unrestrained buying sprees, or foolish business practices

These manic periods can also be associated with major depressive episodes and all the symptoms as described previously, including significant sleep disruptions.

Patients can have full-blown manic episodes as described above, or they can have "hypomanic" periods that are not as extreme and not as long as a manic period. It is classified as bipolar II disorder when patients have hypomania and major depression.

Cyclothymia is mood swings that do not meet the criteria for manic or major depressive disorder but are chronic fluctuating mood periods. Of course, substance abuse can be associated with mood disorders and sleep issues, too.

Sleep issues are found with major depression, dysthymia, bipolar I disorder, bipolar II disorder, cyclothymia, and substance abuse.

Anxiety Disorders

There are a variety of anxiety disorders that can contribute to disrupted sleep, such as generalized anxiety, OCD, PTSD, and panic disorder.

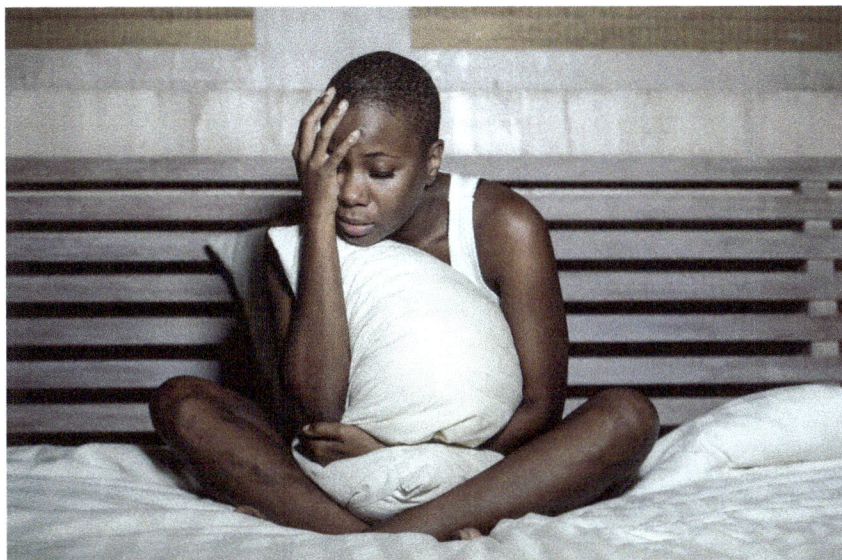

Generalized anxiety disorder (GAD) is excessive anxiety and worry about several events or activities occurring more days than not for at least six months. GAD can be associated with difficulty sleeping, irritability, restlessness, fatigue, muscle aches or soreness, and decreased concentration.

Obsessive compulsive disorder (OCD) involves unwanted, intrusive thoughts or images that persistently recur. They are disruptive and can be time-consuming, and often very frustrating. They are associated with repetitive behaviors or mental acts that the person feels driven to do in an attempt to avoid obsessive thoughts or fears. Obsessive thinking can be very intrusive and about anything, including sleep issues, but it can also be about germs, counting or checking things, religious preoccupations, sexual thoughts or images, etc. The obsessive thoughts and rituals of OCD can disrupt sleep, leading to initial insomnia, frequent awakenings, and disrupted sleep quality.

Post-traumatic stress disorder (PTSD) is a disorder following a traumatic event or situation the patient is a part of or witnesses or hears about, causing alterations in cognition or mood associated with intense fear, helplessness, or horror. Common causes include sexual abuse, military exposure, domestic violence, car accidents, mass shootings, floods, terror attacks, near-death experiences, witnessing death, life-threatening events for children, and events seen by emergency service personnel. These exposures are causative of intrusive thoughts about the event, avoidance, flashbacks, nightmares, distress if exposed to similar situations, isolation, restricted range of affect, insomnia, irritability or mood swings, concentration/memory issues, hypervigilance, and an exaggerated startle response.

The ICD-11 (Organization, 2019/2021) added criteria for a subtype of this disorder called "complex PTSD" of mistaken self-blame, persistent negative mood, irritation/aggression, and impulsive or self-destructive behavior.

The above symptoms can contribute to trouble sleeping, fragmented sleep, and non-restorative sleep for extended periods of time.

"A ruffled mind makes a restless pillow."

~ Charlotte Brontë

Panic disorder is recurrent unexpected panic attacks associated with palpitations, accelerated heart rate, sweating, trembling/shaking, shortness of breath or smothering sensations, chest pain, nausea or GI upset, dizziness or lightheadedness, numbness or tingling, chills or flushing, feelings of unreality, and fears of dying or losing control. Not all of these symptoms must be present at one time to be diagnosed with this disorder. The DSM-5 criteria require four symptoms or more for the diagnosis. These episodes can even occur at night, and when they do, they are called "nocturnal panic attacks." Anxiety, frustration, and fear associated with panic attacks can lead to insomnia and even depression.

Sometimes, sleep paralysis is wrongly diagnosed as nocturnal panic attacks. Sleep paralysis can occur as an independent disorder or be a part of the narcolepsy spectrum. Sleep paralysis is waking and briefly feeling as if your body is paralyzed and you cannot speak. This will be discussed more in Chapter 11 on sleep disorders.

Substance Abuse

Sometimes chronic insomnia can lead to substance abuse, sometimes substance abuse leads to insomnia, and sometimes both factors are at play at the same time.

Alcohol use and nicotine use (even in moderation) can cause sleep disruption and will be discussed in a later chapter. Still, smoking and drinking alcohol are so common we may forget about them as possibly contributing to sleep disruption.

Attempting detox or withdrawal from alcohol, nicotine, or other substances of abuse can certainly play havoc with sleep.

Grau-Lopez et al. in *Frontiers in Psychiatry* (2020) reported that they studied 481 patients receiving pharmacological and psychotherapeutic treatments for detoxification. Insomnia was reported in 66.5%, with sleep-maintenance insomnia being the most common complaint. A higher prevalence of sleep-onset insomnia was seen with alcohol and cannabis use, and increased sleep-maintenance problems were seen with cocaine and heroin use. Independent risk factors for insomnia were identified as polysubstance abuse, female gender, comorbid anxiety disorders, and prior admissions for detoxification. Insomnia was more common early in substance withdrawal, and 57.8% of alcohol users and 56.6% of polysubstance users had issues with insomnia. Patients with a history of polysubstance use were 2.85 times more likely to suffer from insomnia, and those with anxiety disorders were 2.02 times more likely to have insomnia.

A previous study of theirs (Grau-López et al., 2020) found that 84.3% of addicted patients had insomnia during the active consumption of substances.

Also, insomnia is a significant risk factor in relapses for both alcohol disorders and illegal substance use. It, therefore, should be aggressively addressed with non-addicting medications and therapeutic interventions such as cognitive behavioral therapy for insomnia, sleep restriction therapy, progressive muscle relaxation, sleep hygiene, mindful meditation, exercise, and other techniques described later in this book.

In summary, so many mental health issues are associated with sleep disruption. You need sleep to heal from whatever problem is causing mental strain, and the lack of sleep can cause mental health issues, so prioritize your sleep and your mental health! Mental health matters!

"Also, I could finally sleep. And this was the real gift because when you cannot sleep, you cannot get yourself out of the ditch—there's not a chance."

~ *Elizabeth Gilbert in Eat, Pray, Love*

Chapter 7

What and When You Eat and Drink Matters!

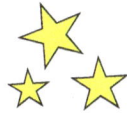

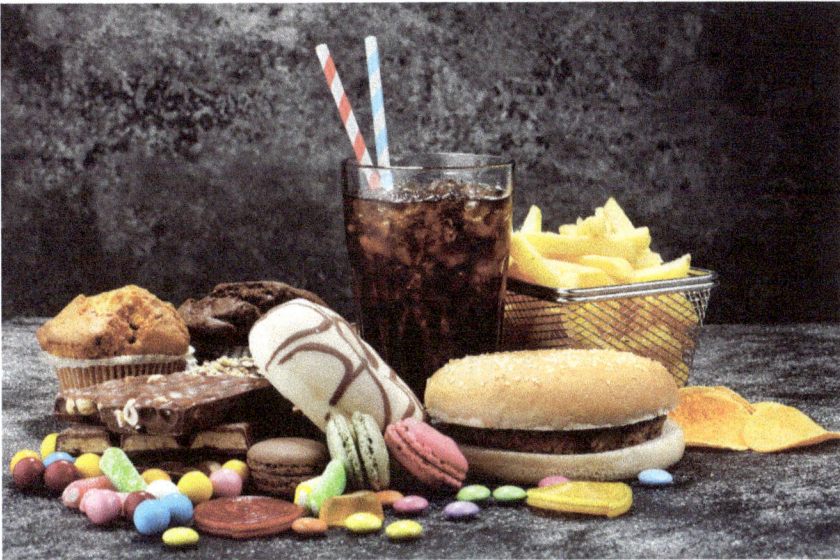

⭐⭐⭐

Increased Weight and Sleep

Let me take a minute to discuss sleep and weight. Even if you don't have sleep apnea or snoring, being overweight can influence your sleep. Even a little weight loss can help with reflux symptoms, breathing, pain, discomfort, arthritis, metabolism, asthma, and mood.

Being overweight increases the risk of developing sleep disorders and having a sleep disorder can increase your risk of being overweight. So, sleep and weight issues are bidirectional.

Not getting enough sleep can increase weight issues! In an interesting article on *Web*MD from April 11, 2024, by Mary Jo Dilanardo (2024) called "The Connection Between Sleep and Obesity," she described the relationship between appetite and sleep. She reported the following:

> Two hormones in your body help control your appetite. Leptin tells your body when you're full. Ghrelin, on the other hand, tells your brain that you're hungry. Like some other hormones, how you get them is related to your sleep/wake cycle, also known as the circadian cycle.
>
> When you don't get enough sleep, your leptin levels go down. So, your brain signals that you're hungry even though you don't need to eat. At the same time, your ghrelin levels go up, so you feel hungry. When you feel those hunger pangs, you're more likely to grab food that's high in fat and calories instead of something healthy.

She also discussed the concept of "the fourth meal" occurring because the longer you are awake, the more time you have to eat, leading to consuming excessive calories in the evening after dinner time. Eating late at night increases weight, creating a vicious cycle.

Not getting enough sleep is also associated with decreased exercise and activity, which can contribute to weight gain or failure to lose weight.

Being overweight can cause osteoarthritis, which can disrupt sleep, increase pain, limit exercise, and create a cycle of sleep/weight issues.

Being overweight can increase gastroesophageal reflux symptoms, which can disrupt sleep, and sleep apnea, which can in turn increase GERD symptoms. Eating heavy meals, spicy foods, or excessive liquids at night can also increase reflux symptoms and disrupt sleep.

So, as you can see, your weight, eating late, increased reflux issues, decreased sleep, an increased risk of apnea, upper airway resistance, and snoring can all disrupt sleep.

Being overweight certainly complicates sleep and sleep disorders, which can lead to sleep disruption, which increases appetite and leads to increased weight. So, the point is to avoid eating and drinking late at night. Work on weight loss and increased exercise. It will help with your sleep (and your weight)!

Alcohol and Sleep

Alcohol use can disrupt your sleep, decrease the quality of your sleep, increase apnea, increase awakenings during sleep, and lead to chronic sleep problems. All of the above symptoms can lead some people to drink more alcohol to try to sleep better, creating an unending cycle of disruption.

As discussed in the previous chapter, while some may think alcohol helps them get to sleep faster, it can cause insomnia and difficulty staying asleep, disrupt your sleep cycles, decrease REM sleep, increase the lighter stage 1 NREM sleep, and cause fragmented, non-restorative sleep.

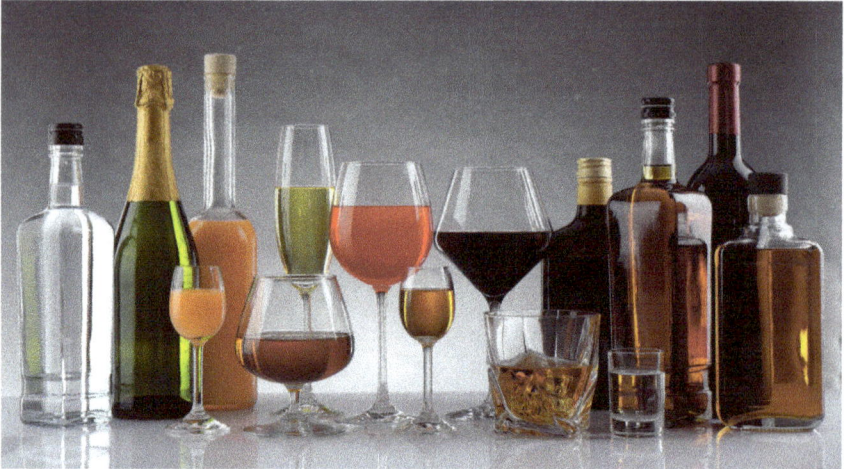

Alcohol can act as a diuretic, increasing nocturia (frequent bathroom trips at night), which also disrupts sleep and leads to an increase in the lighter stages of sleep.

The Sleep Foundation website (sleepfoundation.org) has an article called "Alcohol and Sleep" from May 7, 2024, by Lucy Bryan and Dr. Abhinav Singh, with a great table called "Will a Small Amount of Alcohol Affect My Sleep?" I suggest you look it up. In it, they report that even small amounts can disrupt sleep somewhat.

- **Low** amounts of alcohol decreased sleep quality by **9.3%.**
  - o Defined as less than two drinks for men and **less than one** for women.
- **Moderate** amounts of alcohol decreased sleep quality by **24%**.
  - o Defined as **approximately two drinks** for men and one drink for women.
- **High** amounts of alcohol decreased sleep quality by 39.2%.
  - o Defined as **more than two drinks** for men and **more than one** for women.

An article by He, Hasler, and Chakravorty entitled "Alcohol and Sleep-Related Problems" (2019) discussed a link between alcohol use and insomnia, abnormalities of circadian sleep rhythms, an overall short sleep duration, increased breathing-related sleep issues and oxygen desaturations, evening chronotypes, and the development of "complex insomnia phenotypes." So, alcohol use and sleep have a complex relationship!

Alcohol can:

- Lead to increased nightmares and vivid dreams
- Increase restless legs symptoms
- Increase snoring and worsening of sleep apnea
- Cause nocturia (going to the bathroom during the night) or enuresis (bedwetting)
- Contribute to sleep fragmentation
- Withdrawal from alcohol is also associated with insomnia

It is recommended that you avoid alcohol three to four hours before bedtime to avoid sleep disruption.

Caffeine and Sleep

Caffeine can cause anxiety, irritability, and insomnia. It can be associated with palpitations, panic attacks, tachycardia, increased sweating, and irritability. At higher doses, it can even cause fogginess and decrease the ability to concentrate. Caffeine is a stimulant used by many to increase alertness in the morning. It takes roughly 30 minutes to be effective but can stay in your system for over five to six hours. It may not continue to have the same level of alerting qualities at five to six hours out, but it can reduce sleep and sleep quality if used too close to sleep.

"I love you in that place between coffee and sleep."

~ *Atticus,* The Dark Between Stars

Data posted on the Sleep Foundation website (sleepfoundation. org) from about 160,000 profiles shows that roughly 88% of people who regularly consume caffeine in the afternoon report at least one sleep problem. They report that caffeine makes them fall asleep later, sleep fewer hours overall, and makes their sleep less satisfying. Additionally, it decreases the deep, slow wave sleep they achieve and can lead to feeling unrefreshed the next day.

A 2023 article by Gardiner et al. (2023) in *Sleep Medicine Reviews* was a systematic review and meta-analysis of 24 studies on the effects of caffeine and night-time sleep. This report said that caffeine consumption reduced total sleep time by 45 minutes, increased sleep onset latency (the time to fall asleep) by nine minutes, and increased wakefulness after sleep by 12 minutes. All of this led to a decrease in sleep efficiency of 7% (remember that the definition of normal sleep efficiency is equal to or greater than 85%). Their report indicated increased lighter stages of sleep and less of the deeper stages of NREM sleep, which we feel is more restorative. The amount and timing of the final caffeine dose reduced total sleep time. They recommend consuming coffee at least 8.8 hours before bedtime to avoid reductions in total sleep time.

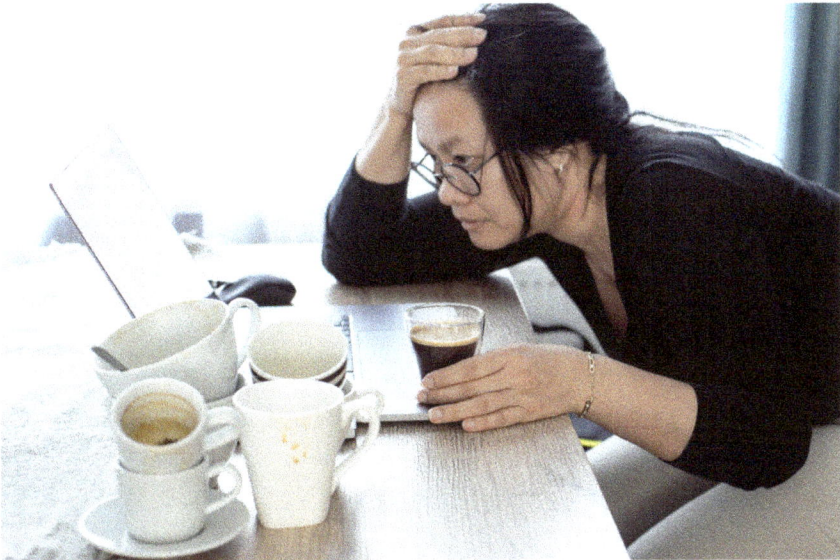

I once had a patient come to my office for an evaluation of insomnia, and she sat a 20 oz Monster Energy drink on my desk. It was about 3:30 PM when she came in. She also suffered from a great deal of anxiety and was drinking up to five to six Monster Energy drinks each day to help her function. As each Monster Energy drink has 79.2 mg of caffeine, and caffeine can stay in your system for several hours. This was a contributing factor to both her insomnia and anxiety. She had various reasons for her insomnia, but she had inadvertently added another one by adding Monster drinks on top of the soft drinks she consumed. This can become a vicious cycle.

The Insomnia/Caffeine Cycle

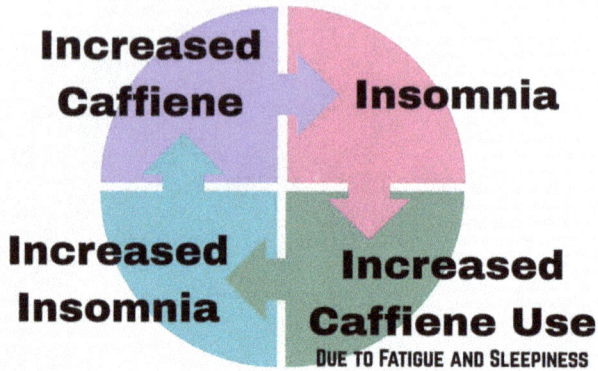

Increased Caffiene → **Insomnia**

Increased Insomnia ← **Increased Caffiene Use**
DUE TO FATIGUE AND SLEEPINESS

Caffeine can be found in:

- Coffee
- Tea
- Soft drinks
- Chocolate and hot chocolate
- Decaffeinated coffee and tea
- Snack bars or candy bars
- Supplements
- Kombucha fermented tea
- Matcha and yerba mate teas
- Workout drinks and energy drinks

Online data suggests some nutritional or energy bars may contain caffeine up to 50 mg to 100 mg or even 250 mg in those marketed as energy bars. For example, Clif Bar's Cool Mint Chocolate with Caffeine has 49 mg of caffeine per bar. "Wake Up!" Bars contain up to 350 mg of plant-based caffeine. "Eat Your Coffee" caffeinated energy bars contain 80 mg of caffeine.

Work-out drinks may also contain caffeine, such as Zevia Zero Calorie Energy Drink, which has 120 mg of organic caffeine per can. Clean Cause Yerba Mate Energy Drink has 160 mg of caffeine, Celsius Energy Drink has 200 mg of caffeine, Uptime Premium Energy Drink has 142 mg of caffeine, Focus Aid Brain Boost Low-Calorie Drink has 100 mg of caffeine, Throne Sport Coffee has 150 mg of caffeine, Sambazon Organic Amazon Energy Low Calorie has 120 mg of caffeine, and Alani Nu Sugar-Free Energy Drink has 200 mg of caffeine.

Red Bull energy drink has 74.8 mg of caffeine, Full Throttle energy drink has 76.8 mg, and Monster energy drink has 79.2 mg.

These are just a few of the options out there. So, you get the point. If you have a couple of these with your evening workout, you have just bought yourself a ticket to insomnia. It creates an endless cycle.

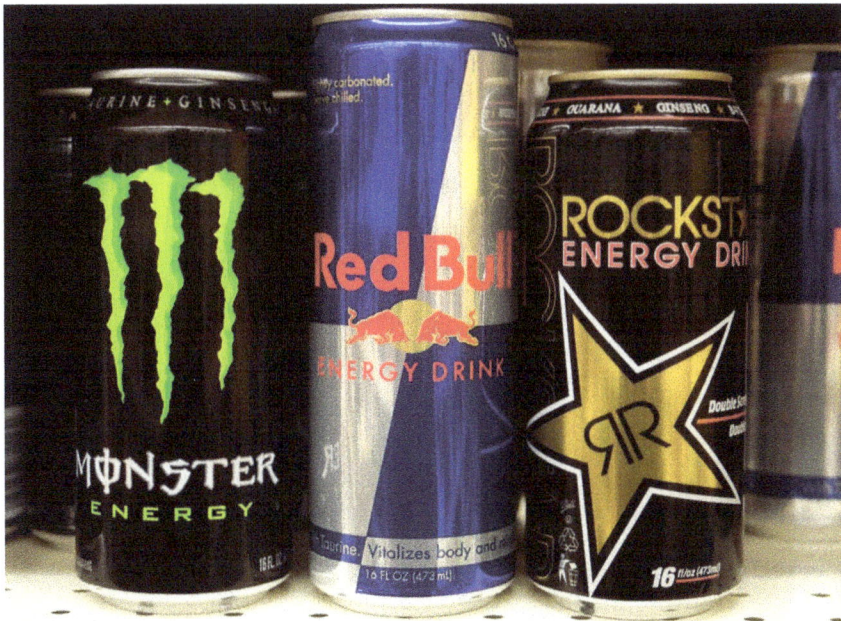

Let's talk about the designer coffees we all love. Driving through for coffee before your afternoon class, drinking a large coffee on your way home from work, and grabbing a large coffee at lunch may all contribute to anxiety and, later on, to insomnia. While they are alerting in the short run, you may pay the price later that night with the inability to wind down and sleep.

Starbucks standard K-cup pods have 130 mg of caffeine on average, and the Starbucks 2X pods have 260 mg. Reportedly, their in-store Venti Blonde Roast brewed coffee contains as much as 475 mg of caffeine! (lifeboostcoffee.net).

Their Venti Medium Roast has 410 mg of caffeine, Trenta Vanilla Sweet Cream Cold Brew has 320 mg, and the medium Clover brewed coffee in Venti size has 445 mg. Blonde Roast has 360 mg, Pike Place 310 mg, Nitro Cold Brew 280 mg, and Dark Roast 260 mg.

I am not singling out Starbucks; they are so widespread nationwide that they provide a reasonable frame of reference for this discussion. My favorite, Chai Tea Latte, still has 95 mg of caffeine.

A small coffee at Dunkin' Donuts has 180 mg of caffeine, and an extra-large has up to 330 mg.

5-hour Energy Extra Strength has 70 mg of caffeine per ounce.

An article called "Caffeine Effects on Sleep Taken 0, 3, or 6 Hours Before Going to Bed" (Drake et al., 2013) found that even a moderate dose of caffeine (400 mg) 6 hours before bed can disrupt sleep.

As reported by Zwyghuizen-Doorenbos et al., tolerance to caffeine's alerting effects develops quickly, which often leads to increased caffeine use (1990). Sepkowitz reported that there may be tolerance to the alerting impact but not the sleep side effects of caffeine (2013).

The sleep "sandwich" effect discussed by O'Callaghan, Muurlink, and Reid (2018) reported that although there are benefits to caffeine, which enhances performance, the withdrawal leads to cognitive, emotional, and behavioral deficits and possibly increases accidents. They proposed that caffeine interrupts sleep, interfering with daytime performance, leading to increased caffeine use and creating a vicious cycle. Their point was that caffeine could be used for side-effect mitigation rather than just performance enhancement.

Just think about how the popularity of caffeine use in adolescents has grown over the years and the available coffee shops on every corner. Orbeta et al. (2006) studied 15,686 American adolescents. They revealed that those who used caffeine heavily during the day were likely to be more tired than those who reported low caffeine use and they had difficulty sleeping. Their report stated that the primary source of caffeine in adolescents was soft drinks, but these days, many adolescents also consume large amounts of designer coffee and energy drinks.

As discussed, chronic and/or excessive use of caffeine may cause a "crash" after the caffeine wears off, reinforcing the need for more caffeine due to drowsiness, headaches, decreased concentration, or irritability during withdrawal. The timing of caffeine use can undoubtedly be an issue, too.

Generally, you should avoid caffeine for at least eight hours before sleep.

If you want to drink coffee in the afternoon, use decaffeinated or at least ½ decaf and ½ regular coffee. Try herbal or noncaffeinated tea. Better yet sometimes, when you are sleepy or sluggish, you are dehydrated and need water. Drink a bottle of water and see if you don't feel more refreshed and energetic.

Nicotine and Sleep

Nicotine is a stimulant and can cause a rapid release of hormones that increase respiration, blood pressure, and heart rate. Nicotine can also affect your sleep. It can cause initial insomnia, decrease sleep quality, and decrease your total sleep time.

Smokers are almost 50% more likely to experience issues with their sleep. This includes those who smoke cigarettes, vape, and use other tobacco products.

Vaping can decrease stage 3 NREM slow-wave sleep.

Nicotine causes increased time to fall asleep, frequent awakenings, and less time in deep restorative sleep.

Nicotine can increase snoring, OSA, and parasomnias (increased movements or vocalizations such as sleepwalking, sleep talking, or night terrors).

Nunez et al. (2021) studied 1007 smokers and nonsmokers in the Philadelphia area. They found that smoking was associated with increased insomnia severity and shorter sleep duration, especially with night-time smoking.

So, try to avoid nicotine four hours before bedtime, and if using nicotine replacement products, stop one hour before bedtime.

Try just the breathing techniques of smoking without a cigarette.

Fluid and Food Intake and Sleep

Don't drink late! This includes water, milk, soft drinks, juice, and the caffeine and alcohol mentioned above. Increased fluids before bedtime can cause frequent bathroom trips and increased GERD. Some drinks may cause blood sugar fluctuations, interfering with sleep.

Small amounts of water before bed may help prevent dehydration, but too much can cause increased awakenings and nocturia. Get enough fluids during the day to avoid dehydration. I recommend drinking a glass of water just as you wake up to help rehydrate, possibly boost your metabolism, hydrate your skin, increase your energy, and improve your cognition.

I drink a glass of water with my coffee each morning and one at lunch to help get enough water throughout the day.

Regarding juice, a small amount of tart cherry juice, which has natural melatonin, has been reported to help with sleep. However, too much has a high sugar content and can also increase bathroom trips.

Some fruits like bananas, berries, kiwis, cherries, and pineapples have melatonin and are good bedtime snacks.

Oatmeal, whole wheat toast, avocado, and Greek yogurt are also good nighttime snacks. Eggs, containing tryptophan, melatonin, and vitamin D, are another good option.

More acidic juices and spicy foods can increase gastroesophageal reflux, possibly increase apnea, and cause heartburn. The capsaicin in spicy food can increase your body temperature, making it harder for you to sleep.

High-salt foods before bedtime can increase your blood pressure.

High-sugar snacks can cause an increase in blood sugar and insulin levels and disrupt your sleep.

High-fat and high-protein meals may take longer to break down if eaten before bedtime, as your digestive system is already slowed during sleep.

Consider what you eat and drink before bedtime to promote healthy sleep.

The 3-2-1 Principle

This idea about sleep recommendations has been floating around for a long time, and I am not sure who first coined the term or principle. Most recently, sleep psychologist Michael Breus was on the *Today* show and recommended that individuals stop drinking alcohol three hours before bed, stop eating two hours before bedtime, and stop drinking fluids one hour before bedtime. These are just general guidelines and should not be something to obsess about, like in orthosomnia. Sometimes, a light snack before bedtime or water to sip on is helpful and refreshing. The point is not to eat a large amount that the stomach cannot digest, which can lead to increased gastroesophageal reflux symptoms at night.

Avoiding drinking alcohol at night and late in the evening is recommended, as it can cause sleep disruptions by increasing apnea, snoring, nightmares, increased bathroom trips during sleep, decreased total sleep time, and decreased REM sleep.

The addition of limiting nicotine would make it the 4-3-2-1 rule by stopping smoking 4 hours before bedtime.

Variations of the 3-2-1 routine include avoiding heavy meals and sugary snacks 3 hours before bedtime. Avoid work or stressful activities 2 hours before bedtime and avoid electronics one hour before bedtime. You get the picture. Prepare, prioritize, and promote better sleep!

The 3-2-1 Principle

3 hours before bedtime,
stop alcohol

2 hours before bedtime,
stop eating

1 hour before bedtime,
limit fluids

Chapter 8

Chronic Pain Matters!

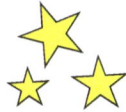

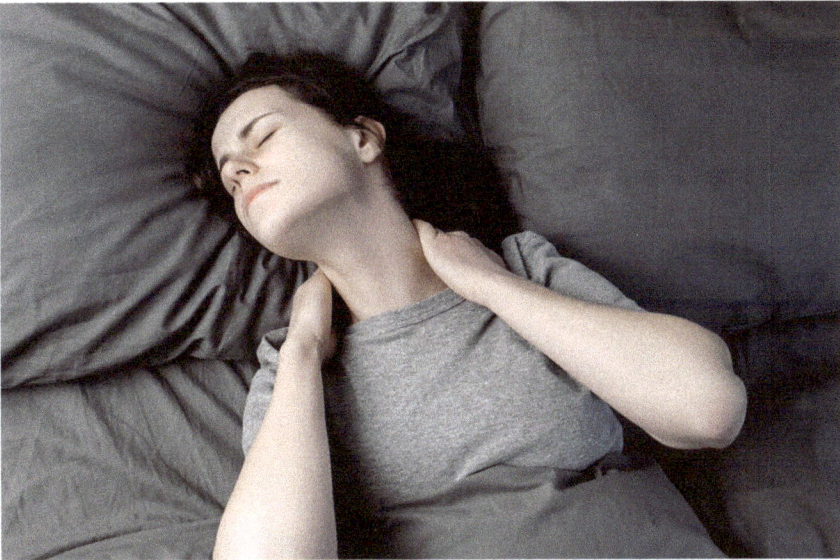

Aggressive pain management at bedtime may help improve sleep quality and quantity. "The Importance of Sleep for People with Chronic Pain: Current Insights and Evidence" (Whale & Gooberman-Hill, 2022) reported that "between 67% and 88% of individuals with chronic pain experience sleep disruption and insomnia, and at least 50% of people with chronic insomnia have chronic pain issues." They reviewed potential nonpharmacological treatments in addition to medications and reported that cognitive behavioral therapy "can provide an equal benefit or be superior to pharmacotherapy."

Cognitive behavioral therapy (CBT) is a type of therapy based on:

1) Looking at unhealthy patterns of thinking and reevaluating them.
2) Looking at unhealthy behavior patterns and taking action to change them.
3) Using problem-solving skills, challenging previous thoughts and behaviors, and creating goals for healthier ways of existence.

CBT has been extensively studied in the treatment of insomnia, as well as other psychiatric disorders and chronic pain.

Their review also highlighted that sleep deprivation is associated with "mental health difficulties, obesity, cancer, type 2 diabetes, heart disease, and many other health conditions." They reported sleep issues in 65% of those with rheumatoid arthritis, 70% with osteoarthritis, and 95% of patients with fibromyalgia.

To improve the quality of life and health, we must simultaneously address pain and sleep.

Sleep and pain may be bidirectional.

The article "Sequential daily relations of sleep, pain intensity, and attention to pain among women with fibromyalgia" (Affleck et al., 1996) discussed the relationship between sleep, pain intensity, and attention to pain among fifty women with fibromyalgia, stating that poorer sleepers tended to report significantly more pain. A night of poor sleep was followed by a substantially more painful day, and a more painful day was followed by a night of poor sleep.

McBeth (2022) looked at sleep disturbance in patients with rheumatoid arthritis and found that optimizing the total sleep time, improving sleep efficiency, decreasing the time to sleep onset, and reducing the variability in total sleep time could all enhance the quality of life in these chronic pain patients.

Studies have also shown that sleep problems can increase the risk of developing fibromyalgia. Mork and Nilsen (2012) completed a longitudinal study of adult females in Norway without fibromyalgia, musculoskeletal pain, or physical impairment. They followed them, comparing those with sleep complaints and those without. They reported a strong dose-dependent association between sleep problems and the risk of developing fibromyalgia and chronic pain.

Van Looveren and associates systematically reviewed the association between sleep and chronic spinal pain (CSP) (2021). They found that chronic lower back pain was associated with more significant sleep disturbances and shorter sleep duration. They reported that "sleep quality, insomnia, and sleep deprivation severity (i.e., sleep quantity), sleep disturbance, and sleepiness were found to be correlated with pain intensity in such a way that higher pain intensity levels were found in CSP patients reporting poorer sleep." They summarized that "sleep seems to be a stronger predictor for the development of CSP than vice versa. Addressing the frequently reported sleep problems in chronic back pain patients is, therefore, a necessary complement to pain management to provide an optimal treatment outcome in this population."

A review article by Finan, Goodin, and Smith (Finan et al., 2013) on the association of sleep and pain reviewed many articles on this association and reported findings such as elevated insomnia symptoms increasing the risk of exacerbating existing headaches or developing new headaches, episodic tension headaches becoming chronic headaches with insomnia, increased risk of developing fibromyalgia after the onset of insomnia, sleep disruption causing increased levels of pain in patients with depression and older adults, as well as a change in next-day affective responses to pain in rheumatoid arthritis and fibromyalgia patients with disrupted sleep. Additionally, they reported that good sleep was helpful in improving the prognosis for those with chronic musculoskeletal pain, tension-type headaches, and migraines.

I could go on with other studies, but you get the point. Good sleep is essential in preventing pain syndromes, modifying pain intensity, regulating the affective responses to pain, and improving quality of life issues relating to chronic pain. Decreased sleep increases pain perception and limitations due to pain. Chronic pain decreases sleep, whereas improved sleep seems to help. It is bidirectional. I believe a good sleep evaluation should be part of any pain evaluation and included in the treatment plan for these patients. All of the sleep treatment recommendations given throughout this book for co-existing disorders present in addition to pain should not be ignored, as anything disrupting sleep can play a role in intensifying the bidirectional nature of sleep and pain.

Using longer half-life pain medications, anti-inflammatory agents, non-hypnotic sleep aids such as Ambien (zolpidem) or Lunesta (eszopiclone), melatonin, melatonin receptor agonists such as Rozerem (ramelteon), muscle relaxers, acetaminophen, antidepressants which help with pain, and meds such as Neurontin (gabapentin) or Lyrica (pregabalin) may help improve pain and ultimately sleep efficiency in chronic pain patients. Caution should be used with high-dose narcotics, muscle relaxers, and hypnotics at bedtime, which may increase sleep-disordered breathing and could be dangerous. Some studies suggest that cannabinoids may be helpful with pain and sleep, but they have not been approved yet for those disorders.

Soaking in a hot bath or taking a hot shower one hour before bedtime may be beneficial as your body temperature, which goes from very hot to cooling off, can promote sleep. Taking a bath and soaking in Epsom salt in a bathtub may help with muscle relaxation and inflammation. Use one to two cups of Epsom salt in the tub. If you cannot get into a bathtub, create an Epsom salt compress by dissolving one cup of Epsom salt in one quart of warm water. Soak a towel in the solution and apply where needed for fifteen to thirty minutes. Light stretching, yoga, meditation, and progressive muscle relaxation (PMR) may be helpful. Progressive muscle relaxation involves tensing and then relaxing muscles, starting at one end of the body and moving towards the other. This behavior is paired with gently and slowly breathing in and out.

Comfort measures such as foam mattress toppers and additional supportive pillow placements may also help. An example would be putting pillows behind your back if you are a side sleeper or between the knees. Creams to rub on joints for joint pain, such as Voltaren® (diclofenac), Blue EMU®, ibuprofen and ketoprofen gels, gabapentin gels, Biofreeze®, or various compounded gels, can also be helpful.

If you are a back sleeper with chronic back pain, place a pillow under your knees and have a supportive pillow under your head to keep your neck aligned with your chest and back. If you are a stomach sleeper with chronic back pain issues, place a pillow under your hips and lower stomach area.

Plantar fasciitis causes dull, aching heel and arch pain due to inflammation in the plantar fascia in your feet. Possible treatments include night splints to maintain the foot in a stretched position, soaking feet in an ice bath or Epson salts, wearing orthotics, using good supportive shoes during the day, and specific pillows to elevate the foot and keep the foot off the bed that can be ordered online to ease foot pain. They even make pillows that elevate from the hip to the ankle area.

In summary, attempt to address chronic pain issues in many ways, including behavioral and pharmacological interventions to improve sleep and aid in pain perception and tolerance.

Chapter 9

Electronics at Night Matter!

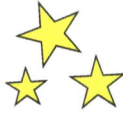

"Some people can't sleep because they have insomnia. I can't sleep because I have internet."

~ Anonymous

Light Effects

Surfing the internet, scrolling on Facebook or Instagram, skipping through TikTok videos, and checking/responding to emails stimulate your brain. Additionally, they do not help with the winding down needed to promote healthy sleep. I recommend that electronics be off at least one hour before bedtime.

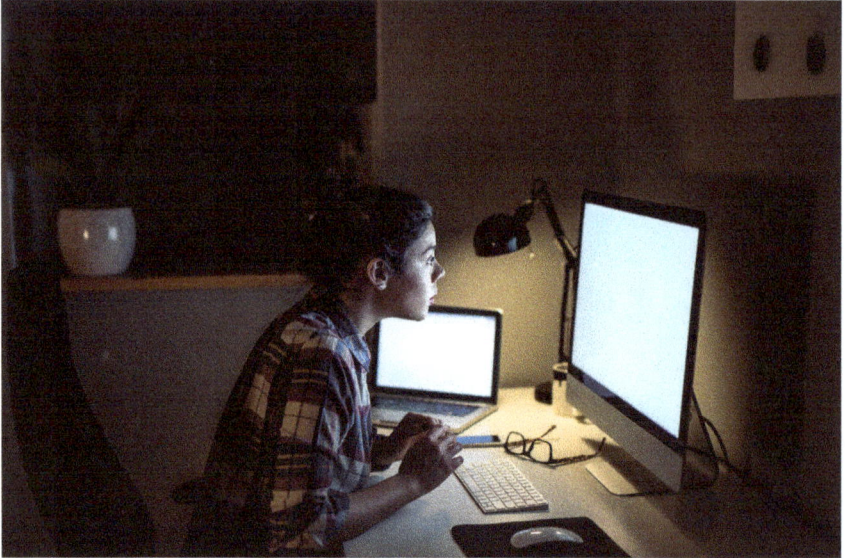

The color of light can affect circadian rhythms. White light during the day can improve mood and alertness. In fact, we often recommend light therapy using a 10,000-lux lamp for depression, especially seasonal affective disorder. It should be used first thing in the morning for 20–30 minutes; you do not need to stare at it. You can read the newspaper or a book, listen to music, eat breakfast, or work while using it.

If sleepy, go to a bright, sunny place or near the light, even on an overcast day. This can help with mood and sleepiness.

Blue light has the most substantial impact on the circadian rhythm and is emitted from computer screens, cell phones, tablets, TVs, and fluorescent bulbs. It suppresses the production of melatonin, which helps regulate sleep.

The CDC National Institute of Occupational Safety and Health (NIOSH) 2020 report (federalregister.gov) states, "Blue light waves come from fluorescent and LED lights and back-lit electronic screens." Exposure to this type of light during sensitive periods can disrupt sleep by making it difficult to fall and stay asleep and cause one to wake up too early.

According to the CDC NIOSH report, red light does not affect circadian rhythms, and using a dim red light at night is better. Yellow and orange light have little effect and can also be used.

So, consider changing your surrounding lights, wearing blue light-blocking glasses, or making other interventions, such as decreasing screen brightness in the evening.

Following Facebook and what appears to be all happy people doing outstanding activities with their perfect families, jobs, cars, and pets can lead to comparison and a sense of "missing out." In fact, this is often called "FOMO," standing for the "fear of missing out," and people with this issue usually check their phones frequently during the day, while socializing with others, before sleep, even waking during sleep to check their phone, if they get up to go to the bathroom at night, and while driving. At the same time, the post is just a snapshot of one moment in time and may not reflect the reality of most people's rather mundane lives. This comparison can lead to anxiety, loneliness, feelings of inadequacy, and frustration.

Playing Candy Crush, Wordle, Minecraft, and other games on your phone or tablet before sleep can be stimulating, alerting, and even anxiety-provoking, not to mention the exposure to blue light.

Waking during sleep to check social media or your phone after falling asleep is very disruptive to obtaining the deeper sleep cycles needed for restorative sleep. The Sleep Foundation "Sleep and Social Media" post by Rob Newsom and Dr. Anis Rehman from December 22, 2023, states that 21% of adults say that they wake up to check their phone during the night, and 70% of people report using social media after getting into bed with 15% spending more than an hour doing so. Newsom and Rehman recommend:

- Make tuning out a habit by having screen-free time every day, perhaps while socializing, around mealtime, and before bed.
- Notice your FOMO (fear of missing out) and learn to cope with feelings of anxiety by trying some relaxation exercises.

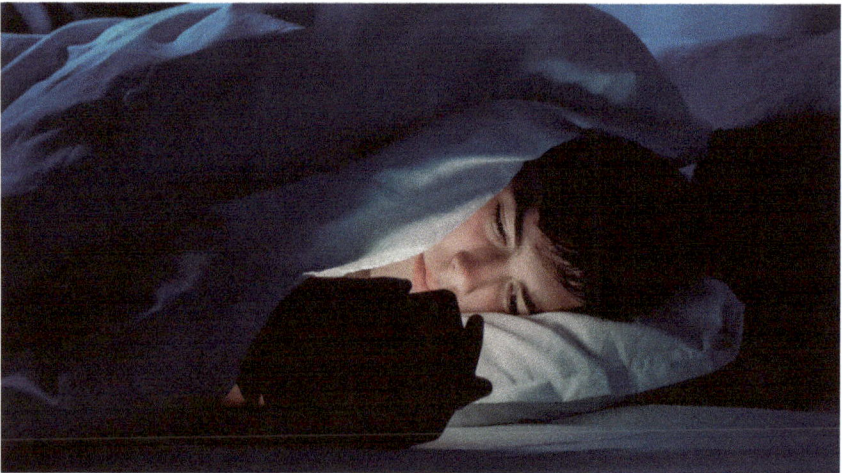

- Silence alerts and notifications.
- Charge your phone in a different room.
- If necessary, see a doctor or counselor. Like any other activity, it can become an obsession.

Gaming is a nocturnal sport for most and is especially common among adolescents and young adults who have a large community of friends locally, across the nation, and sometimes in other countries.

A study by Peracchia and Curico called "Exposure to video games: effects on sleep and on post-sleep cognitive abilities. A systematic review of experimental evidence" (Peracchia & Curcio, 2018) revealed reduced total sleep time, increased sleep onset latency, poor sleep quality, increased fatigue, and reported video games may contribute to decreased cognitive and behavioral activities the next day. It can become its own vicious cycle and lead to the development of delayed sleep phase syndrome or going to bed late and sleeping late each day.

This is not to mention that most serious gamers multitask by playing games, texting, and watching television simultaneously, further increasing mental, visual, and sound stimulation. They also often consume energy drinks while doing so.

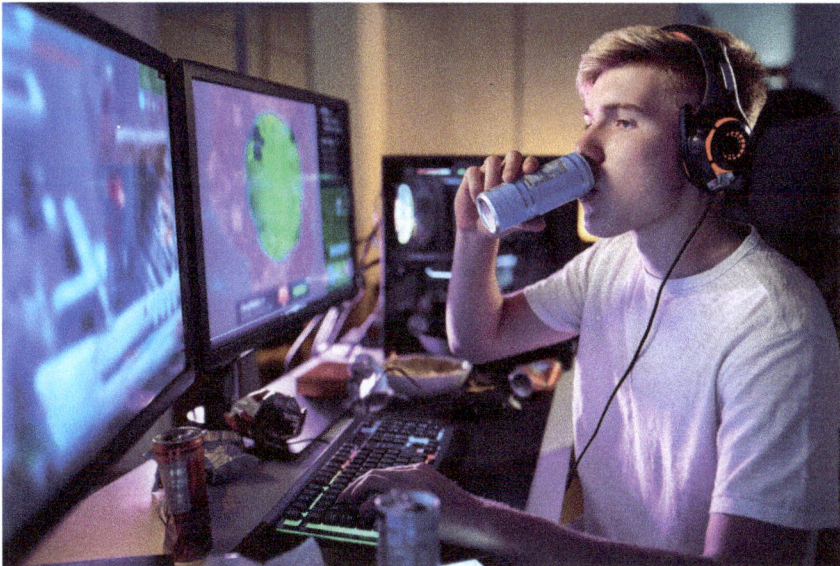

Hanging out in the dark all day and all evening is not good for your mental or physical health. We need light to help set our circadian rhythm and for our mood, energy, cognition, and sleep.

Now, let's talk about some tips for electronics and sleep.

- Plan an electronics time two or three hours before bedtime. Stay in another room to play and set a timer. When the timer goes off, go into your bedroom and relax. Read a book or put a low-stimulating comedy or TV show on to help you wind down. We want you to associate your bed with relaxation, peace, winding down, and sleep.
- Keeping your lights low and volume down while using social media can also be helpful by being less stimulating.
- Silence alerts and notifications during sleep.
- It would be ideal if you could have a designated electronics area outside the bedroom!
- Stop playing video games at least one to two hours before the desired bedtime.
- Another thing to consider is how many hours in a row you spend playing video games...talk about winding you up!! At least schedule a little break, get some fresh air, visit your family, step outside for the sunlight, exercise, or do something else you enjoy!
- Wear blue-light-blocking glasses to decrease blue-light exposure before bedtime, as blue light suppresses melatonin. These can be ordered on the Internet.
- Caffeine consumption while playing video games can also disrupt sleep. Drink water, decaffeinated beverages, or milk, and avoid drinking six to eight sodas or energy drinks each evening while gaming.

Chapter 10

Medications Matter!

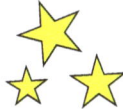

Medications affect everyone differently. For instance, many people take Benadryl (diphenhydramine) to help them sleep. Still, in some patients, it can increase restless leg symptoms and lead to increased initial insomnia, kicking during sleep, and non-restorative sleep. It can also contribute to feeling "hungover" and sleepy the next day. Alternatively, a small dose of this medicine helps others sleep and wake up energetically.

I had one of my patients with significant insomnia complaints who was taking *six* of the 25 mg Benadryl tablets at night because of her inability to sleep...150 mg! What she had actually done was increase her restless legs symptoms dramatically, creating more insomnia, increase her dry mouth and slurred speech to the point others thought she was taking some drugs, and made an extreme "hangover" of daytime sleepiness due to the large quantity of medication she was taking. (Not to mention other side effects of constipation, blurred vision, etc.)

Antidepressants also have various effects on different individuals. Some antidepressants are very sedating and taking them at night can be helpful. For others, antidepressants may be more energizing. Cymbalta (duloxetine), Effexor (venlafaxine), and Pristiq (desvenlafaxine) have been known to increase restless legs symptoms, periodic limb movements, and sleep disruptions in some; to others, they do not interfere with sleep. Wellbutrin (bupropion) is generally a more alerting medication and is given earlier in the day. It can lead to insomnia if taken too late. A newer, often more beneficial combination for resistant depression consists of bupropion and dextromethorphan and is marketed as Auvelity (dextromethorphan-bupropion). It is usually prescribed twice daily, and I recommend it in the morning and at dinnertime.

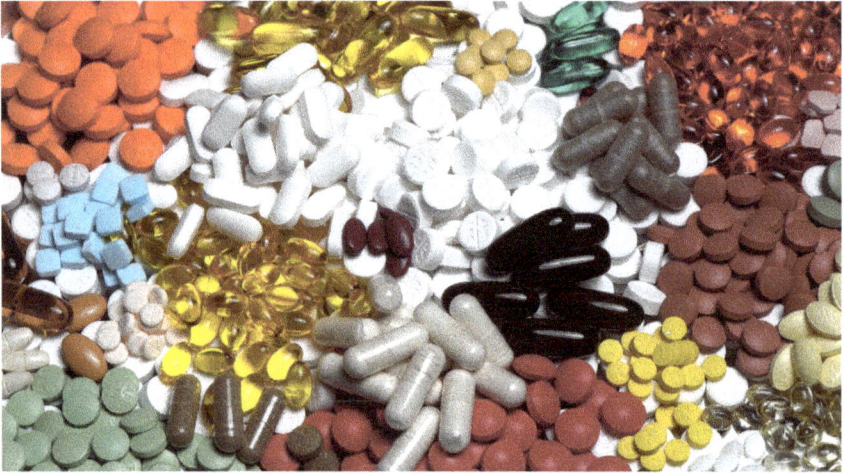

It may be helpful to take many medicines prescribed twice daily in the morning and at dinnertime, instead of morning and nighttime. For example, with medications that have a diuretic component or those that induce nocturia (going to the bathroom at night), taking them in the morning and using them at dinnertime and not bedtime can immediately be beneficial in decreasing sleep disruptions from extra bathroom trips.

I am going to provide you with a list of medications that can increase insomnia, restless legs syndrome, nocturia (frequent bathroom trips), enuresis (urinating during sleep), nightmares, and night terrors. These lists are not exhaustive lists of the medications contributing to these disorders. These are general summaries from internet searches. I suggest you speak with your pharmacist if you have any of these symptoms and are on multiple medications.

Medications Associated with Insomnia

- Stimulants such as Adderall (amphetamine/dextroamphetamine) and Ritalin (methylphenidate)
- Decongestants such as those containing pseudoephedrine and phenylephrine, including Dayquil, Sudafed, Claritin-D, and Allegra-D
- Stimulating antidepressants such as Wellbutrin (bupropion) and Prozac (fluoxetine), and antidepressants that increase restless leg symptoms such as the SNRI antidepressants Cymbalta (duloxetine), Pristiq (desvenlafaxine), and Effexor (venlafaxine)
- Steroids such as Prednisone and Dexamethasone
- Beta blockers such as Inderal (propranolol) and Lopressor (metoprolol)
- Thyroid medication such as higher doses of Synthroid (levothyroxine)
- Diuretics such as Lasix (furosemide) and HCTZ (hydrochlorothiazide)
- Theophylline
- Antiepileptics such as Lamictal (lamotrigine), Topamax (topiramate) and others can increase or decrease sleep
- Antipsychotics
- Diabetes meds such as Metformin
- Pain meds such as the opiates
- Nicotine replacement treatments such as Chantix (varenicline)
- Appetite suppressants

- Caffeine containing medications for headaches such as Excedrin Migraine and Anacin
- Some herbal remedies

Medications That Can Increase Restless Legs Syndrome

- Antihistamines such as Benadryl (diphenhydramine) and Vistaril (hydroxyzine)
- Melatonin and other over-the-counter sleep aids
- Calcium channel blockers such as verapamil and diltiazem
- Antipsychotics such as Haldol (haloperidol), Zyprexa (olanzapine), Risperdal (risperidone) and Seroquel (quetiapine)
- Antinausea meds such as Reglan (metoclopramide) and Compazine (prochlorperazine)
- Antidepressants such as Prozac (fluoxetine), Zoloft (sertraline), Cymbalta (duloxetine), Effexor (venlafaxine) and Remeron (mirtazapine)
- Lithium
- Statin medications such as Lipitor (atorvastatin) or Crestor (rosuvastatin)
- Ultram (tramadol)

Medications Associated with Nightmares, Night Terrors, and Vivid Dreams

- Antidepressants such as Pamelor (nortriptyline), Prozac (fluoxetine), Zoloft (sertraline), Paxil (paroxetine), Sinequan (doxepin), or Elavil (amitriptyline)
- Blood pressure meds such as beta blockers, including Inderal (propranolol), Coreg (carvedilol), Toprol or Lopressor (metoprolol)

- Antipsychotics such as Zyprexa (olanzapine), Seroquel (quetiapine), Risperdal (risperidone), or Clozaril (clozapine)
- Antibiotics and antivirals such as Cipro (ciprofloxacin), Sustiva (efavirenz), Lariam (mefloquine), and Erythromycin
- Sleep aids such as Ambien (zolpidem), Lunesta (eszopiclone), or Sonata (zaleplon)
- Dementia meds such as Aricept (donepezil), Sinemet (carbidopa/levodopa) or Symmetrel (amantadine)
- Stimulants such as Adderall (amphetamine/dextroamphet-amine), Ritalin (methylphenidate), or Provigil (modafinil) or withdrawal from these meds
- Benzodiazepines such as Valium (diazepam), Xanax (alprazolam), Ativan (lorazepam), and Klonopin (clonazepam)
- Beta Blockers such as Inderal (propranolol), Lopressor (metoprolol), or Tenormin (atenolol)
- Narcotics such as morphine, OxyContin (oxycodone), or Vicodin (hydrocodone)
- Statin medications to lower cholesterol
- Melatonin can cause very vivid dreams and sometimes nightmares
- Chantix (varenicline) used to help to stop smoking can cause vivid dreams and nightmares
- Anti-Parkinson's medications and those used for restless legs, such as L-Dopa (levodopa) and Requip (ropinirole) or those used for dementia like Aricept (donepezil), and Exalon (rivastigmine)
- GLP-1 agonists like Ozempic (semaglutide), Wegovy (semaglutide), and Zepbound (tirzepatide)
- Ketamine
- Steroids such as prednisone and methylprednisolone

Medications that can Cause Excessive Daytime Sleepiness

- Opioid pain medications such as oxycodone, hydrocodone, and morphine
- Muscle relaxers such as Amrix (cyclobenzaprine) and Soma (carisoprodol)
- Blood pressure medications such as clonidine
- Antihistamines such as Benadryl (diphenhydramine) and Vistaril (hydroxyzine)
- Sleeping pills such as Restoril (temazepam), Klonopin (clonazepam), Valium (diazepam), Ambien CR (zolpidem), or Lunesta (eszopiclone)
- Antidepressants such as Remeron (mirtazapine), Elavil (amitriptyline), Desyrel (trazodone) and other Tricyclic antidepressants
- Seizure medications like Neurontin (gabapentin), Lyrica (pregabalin), Luminal/Solfoton (phenobarbital)
- Antipsychotics such as Seroquel (quetiapine) or Zyprexa (olanzapine)

Medications Associated with Nocturia (Going to the Bathroom at Night)

- Diuretics such as Lasix (furosemide), Aldactone (spironolactone), and HCTZ (hydrochlorothiazide)
- Blood pressure medications such as calcium channel blockers, ACE Inhibitors, and alpha blockers
- Antidepressants – SSRI's and TCAs such as Lexapro (escitalopram), Prozac (fluoxetine), Paxil (paroxetine), and Effexor (venlafaxine)
- Antipsychotics such as Risperdal (risperidone)
- Mood stabilizers such as Lithium

- Medications for GERD such as Reglan (metoclopramide)
- Dilantin (phenytoin)
- Dementia meds such as Aricept (donepezil), Exelon (rivastigmine), or Namenda (memantine)
- Diabetic medications such as Jardiance (empagliflozin) and Invokana (canagliflozin)
- Long term steroid use such as Prednisone, Hydrocortisone, and Dexamethasone
- Chronic use of NSAIDs such as Advil or Motrin (ibuprofen), Aleve (naproxen) or Aspirin
- Theophylline for COPD

Medications Associated with Enuresis (Bedwetting)

- Diuretics such as Lasix (furosemide), HCTZ (hydrochlorothiazide), and Aldactone (spironolactone)
- Benzodiazepines such as Valium (diazepam), Ativan (lorazepam), or Klonopin (clonazepam)
- Lithium
- Long-term use of steroids such as prednisone, dexamethasone, or hydrocortisone
- Antipsychotics such as Risperdal (risperidone), Seroquel (quetiapine), or Zyprexa (quetiapine)
- Nonsteroidal antiinflammatory drugs (NSAIDs) such as Motrin (ibuprofen) or Aleve (naproxen)
- Cough medications containing dextromethorphan or codeine
- Sleeping pills such as Ambien (zolpidem)
- Estrogen or other HRT and less often progesterone
- Antihistamines and decongestants can cause urinary retention or overflow incontinence
- Blood pressure medications, especially those containing a diuretic

Medications affect everyone differently; a listed medication might not even impact your sleep. Alternatively, other medications may have drastic effects on your sleep. The combination of medicines may be the issue. Consider the possibilities, review with your provider, or talk with your pharmacist to see if adjustments are necessary if you have any of the above symptoms.

Chapter 11

Diagnosing and Treatment of Other Sleep Disorders Matters!

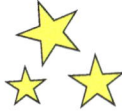

This chapter will discuss many sleep disorders that can disrupt sleep. Some will be more common, like snoring, sleep apnea, sleepwalking, and leg cramps, and others will be more unusual, and you may not even realize they are an actual disorder. Let me start by describing the definition of parasomnias, which are unusual behaviors during sleep, such as talking, acting out a dream, sleepwalking, etc. Parasomnias that occur during REM sleep include nightmares, REM behavior disorder (RBD), and sleep paralysis. Parasomnias that occur during non-REM sleep include night terrors, sleepwalking, and confusional arousals. Other parasomnias include bedwetting, sleep-related groaning, sexsomnia, exploding head syndrome, and sleep-related hallucinations. Parasomnias may be genetic, due to sleep deprivation or an irregular sleep-wake schedule, and, in children, they are often due to sleep-wake cycle immaturity.

Parasomnias have been associated with chronic pain, sleep apnea, narcolepsy, restless legs syndrome, circadian rhythm disorders, and other things that disrupt sleep. Alcohol use, stress, and running a fever may increase their occurrence. Some medications have been reported to lead to parasomnias, such as antihypertensive medications, sedatives, antidepressants, antibiotics, seizure medications, and antipsychotics. We will discuss these and other sleep-related disorders in this chapter.

Sleep Apnea/Snoring

*"Laugh and the world laughs with you,
snore and you sleep alone."*

~ Anthony Burgess

Primary Snoring

As I have said before, not everyone who snores has sleep apnea. Snoring is not always a benign symptom; it is not just something to laugh about. Snoring can be due to weight issues, upper airway obstructions such as nasal polyps, alcohol use before bedtime, nasal congestion/allergies, an elongated uvula (which is the tissue hanging down in the back of your throat), enlarged tonsils, and sleeping on one's back. Snoring can contribute to daytime sleepiness, irritability/anger, nonrestorative sleep, decreased concentration, hypertension, and strokes, even if sleep apnea is absent. Bai et al. (2021) reported snoring is associated with a 46% increased risk of stroke. A sleep study should be initiated to rule out sleep apnea, especially when other medical, mental, academic, or occupational issues are present with snoring.

Treatment recommendations for primary snoring include:

- Losing weight and avoiding further weight gain
- Avoiding alcohol and sedatives before bedtime
- An ENT (ear, nose, and throat) evaluation to rule out reversible causes of airway obstruction
- Aggressive treatment of nasal congestion or allergies
- Over-the-counter snore guards for the nose
- Oral appliances
- Positional therapy to avoid sleeping in the supine position and avoid sleeping flat are often helpful. This can be accomplished with the newer adjustable beds, the use of wedge pillows, extra pillows to sleep on, or elevating the top of the bed and not the bottom of the bed with plywood under the head of the bed.

Sleep Apnea

There are multiple types of sleep apnea.

Obstructive sleep apnea is diagnosed by polysomnography or a home sleep test demonstrating obstructive apneas or hypopnea during sleep associated with snoring, snorting, witnessed respiratory pauses, daytime sleepiness, fatigue, headaches, brain fog, nocturia, sexual dysfunction, issues with mood, hypertension, and a whole host of other medical disorders. Not all of these symptoms have to be present to diagnose this disorder. Being overweight, having a large neck size, using alcohol in the evenings before sleep, smoking, and problems with gastroesophageal reflux can all increase the risk of sleep apnea.

Central sleep apnea is apnea that is due to medications such as opiates, congestive heart failure, higher altitudes, and in those with neurologic conditions such as strokes, tumors, or trauma and lesions to the brainstem. A variety of issues can lead to central sleep apnea, even renal failure. Symptoms include sleepiness, insomnia, and frequent awakenings. While it sounds similar to obstructive sleep apnea, their presentations on the PSG sleep study appear different, symptoms may be different, their treatments can vary, and the usual causes are different, but they can cooccur. When they do, it is called "**complex sleep apnea**."

Central sleep apnea results from a lack of the drive to breathe, while airway issues cause obstructive sleep apnea.

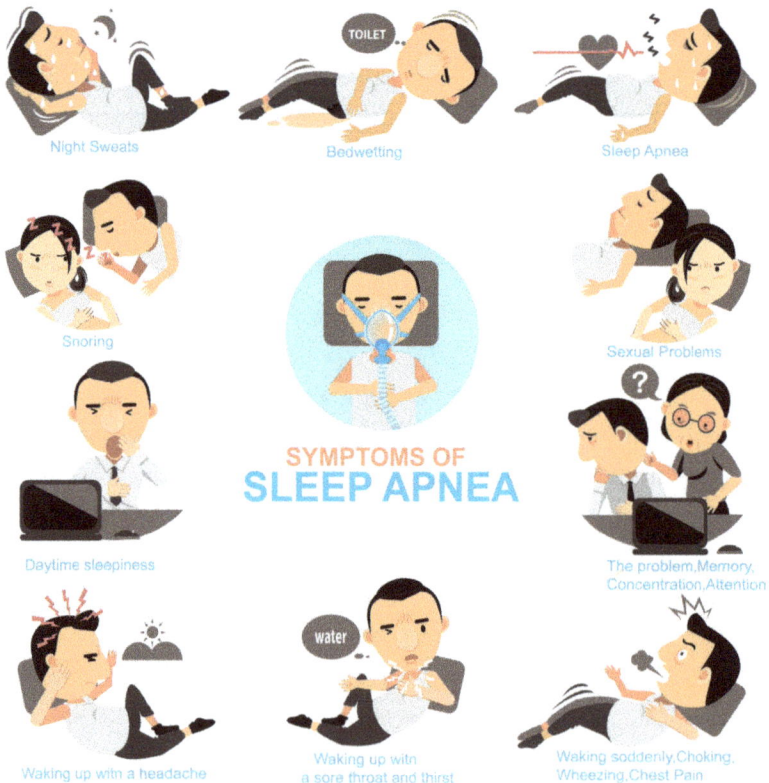

SYMPTOMS OF
SLEEP APNEA

Symptoms of sleep apnea can vary between individuals. It can result in daytime sleepiness, snoring, safety issues due to sleepiness while driving, morning headaches, night sweats, sexual dysfunction, and memory or concentration problems, leading to academic or occupational difficulties. Apnea can cause frequent bathroom trips or even bedwetting. It can lead to depression or irritability, relationship issues, and an increased risk of other health problems or complications with anesthesia.

Apnea treatment often includes CPAP (continuous positive airway pressure), oral appliances to help keep the airway open, surgery, and medications. FDA-approved medications for sleep apnea's excessive daytime sleepiness include Provigil (modafinil), Nuvigil (armodafinil), and Sunosi (solriamfetol). Sometimes, stimulants are also used. A different kind of CPAP is often used for central sleep apnea, but it is essential to treat the underlying cause when possible.

A newer treatment for obstructive apnea is *Inspire,* a surgically implanted device that stimulates the hypoglossal nerve, controls the tongue muscle, and helps to keep the airway open. Inspire treatment is used in those not tolerant of CPAP and those with moderate to severe apnea. It is not used in central or complex apnea.

Surgical options for sleep apnea include removing the tonsils, trimming the uvula and possibly the soft palate, repairing a deviated septum, removing nasal polyps, reducing the size of the nasal turbinate, and even moving the upper and lower jaw forward to make the airway larger. In very extreme cases, a tracheostomy is used.

Treatment also includes:

- Aggressive treatment of allergies, colds, and nasal congestion
- Reviewing medications/situations that may be contributing, such as avoiding alcohol, muscle relaxers, sedatives, and smoking before bedtime
- Avoiding large meals before bedtime
- Positional therapy, as described previously, is used to avoid sleeping in the flat supine position by using wedge pillows, adjustable beds, elevating the head of the bed by 30 degrees by using plywood under the top of the bed and not the bottom part of the bed, or by using a customized nightshirt with a pocket on the back for tennis balls to avoid sleeping in the supine position.
- In mild to moderate OSA cases, oral appliances are helpful and can be used with or without CPAP. These are best supervised by a dentist familiar with this treatment rather than just over-the-counter styles.
- An ENT evaluation is essential to rule out any reversible causes of airway obstruction.
- Weight loss and avoiding further weight gain are helpful with obstructive sleep apnea. Even a weight change of ten to fifteen pounds may increase apnea and require CPAP adjustments.
- Most recently, Zepbound (tirzepatide), the diabetes medicine sometimes used for weight loss, has been approved for adults with moderate-to-severe obstructive sleep apnea and obesity. This is an exciting update for the sleep world! One must keep in mind with this treatment, as weight loss progresses an adjustment in CPAP settings may be necessary, and with significant weight loss, CPAP may no longer be required.

- If prescribed CPAP for the treatment of apnea, some behavioral interventions that can help obtain successful use are: A desensitization program with the CPAP mask, in which the patient wears the mask not attached to the machine while watching TV or listening to music to adjust to the mask's feel before adding the pressure from the CPAP machine. This can be done for a few days before even starting with CPAP.
- Having realistic expectations about the amount of time CPAP must be used. The ultimate goal is to use it all night, but initially, working up to four to five hours of use each night would be considered successful. It is a process, and it sometimes takes time to adjust.
- With considerable anxiety about using CPAP and possibly even performance anxiety, we may use a trial of a nonbenzodiazepine sleep medicine to aid with anxiety and sleep.
- Nasal steroid sprays, allergy meds, and oral decongestants may help to clear the airway and promote greater ease of use.
- Contour CPAP pillows are available online for side or stomach sleepers to aid with CPAP use.
- Sometimes, we must try several masks to find the best fit.
- Humidifying air and using a "ramp" of 20 minutes of slowly increasing CPAP pressure to allow patients time to adjust to higher pressures may improve tolerability.
- If CPAP is still not tolerated, we can switch to another treatment called BIPAP (bilevel positive airway pressure), which uses two different pressures during inhaling and exhaling.

With sleep apnea, safety issues should be addressed, such as driving or other dangerous activities when suffering from excessive daytime sleepiness. The wake-promoting medications Sunosi

(Solriamfetol), Provigil (modafinil), and Nuvigil (armodafinil) or stimulants mentioned previously may be helpful in these situations, even if only taken on an as-needed basis.

Patients with sleep apnea must also know that apnea can be associated with perioperative complications. Patients should always tell surgeons and anesthesia personnel about their apnea before any surgical procedure. Also, informing the primary care provider is essential, as apnea can be associated with many other health problems, and certain medications can increase apnea.

Narcolepsy

I love treating narcolepsy and teaching others about the disorder. My first book, *Wake Up Sleepy Head! Diagnosing, Understanding, and Navigating Narcolepsy* was released at the end of 2023. I will share parts of the book here. For further review, it is available on Amazon, other book websites, and my website, www.drdebrastultz. com.

Narcolepsy is excessive daytime sleepiness and an irrepressible need to sleep or the habit of falling asleep unintentionally. Hypersomnia or excessive daytime sleepiness is the **only** symptom necessary for the diagnosis.

Symptoms associated with narcolepsy include:

- Excessive daytime sleepiness
- Cataplexy
- Sleep paralysis
- Hypnogogic hallucinations
- Disrupted nocturnal sleep
- Brain fog (concentration, memory, and focus issues)

Cataplexy is any brief intermittent muscle weakness that occurs with emotion while a person is awake. It results from an intrusion of REM sleep during wake, which can cause muscle weakness or even complete collapse. It can be subtle or more extreme and can be brief or last for more extended periods. It is present in about 65–75% of patients with narcolepsy and can be overlooked for many years before being recognized and diagnosed.

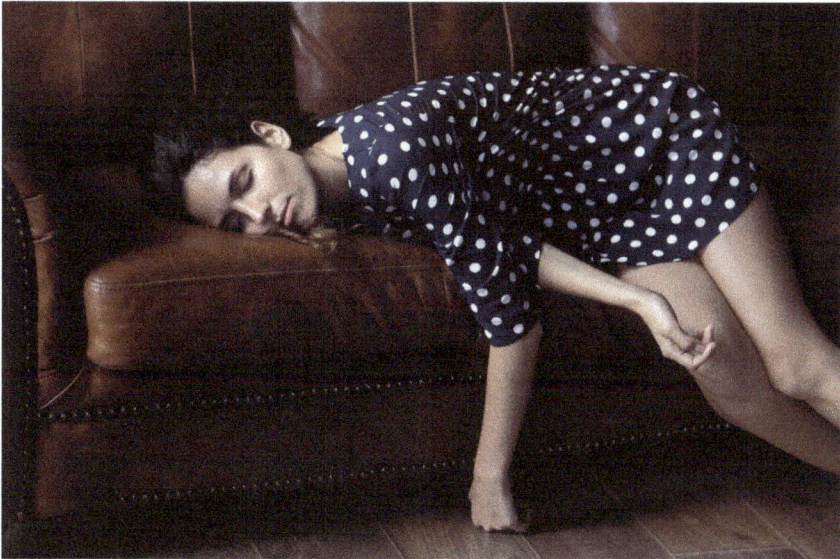

Sleep paralysis occurs when someone wakes up and briefly feels paralyzed. Their mind is awake, but their body is still asleep, and they have the muscle paralysis of REM sleep. They cannot speak or move anything besides their eyes, and their diaphragm continues to regulate breathing.

Hypnogogic and hypnopompic hallucinations are sensory perceptions of auditory, visual, tactile, sensory, or other unusual sensations that occur when going to or coming from sleep. They usually happen when going to sleep and can be experienced as hearing music, seeing things, sensing a presence in the room, or as if someone is touching them, all while this is not happening around them.

Brain fog is the concentration, memory, attention, and focus problems patients complain of with narcolepsy, often describing it "as if I am walking through sludge."

Disrupted nocturnal sleep: Patients with narcolepsy are chronically sleepy but rarely sleep well. Their sleep is often very fragmented. They go into REM sleep quickly, have less slow wave stage 3 NREM sleep, and most of their sleep is very light and unrefreshing.

There are two different types of narcolepsy:

- Narcolepsy type 1 with cataplexy and/or hypocretin deficiency
- Narcolepsy type 2 without cataplexy

So, cataplexy differentiates between the two types. Hypocretin is a substance in cerebral spinal fluid and aids in diagnostic clarification but is not frequently ordered or completed.

Presentations of cataplexy include:

- Head dropping and the neck giving way
- Drooping eyelids
- Blurred vision
- Double vision
- Trouble focusing
- Raised eyebrows
- Slurred or garbled speech
- Stuttering
- Sagging jaw
- Tongue protrusion
- Unusual facial weakness or movement

- Smile disruption
- Shoulder weakness
- Arm weakness
- Hand weakness and frequently dropping things (like cell phones)
- Inability to write or frequently dropping a pencil or pen
- Clumsiness or tripping over their feet
- Unexplained falls
- Leg or ankle weakness
- Knee buckling or knee unlocking
- Trembling of the knees from weakness alternating with contractions
- Complete collapse
- Feeling as if their body is going limp
- Slumping
- Eyes fluttering
- Slurring speech or fading out of speech
- Muscle jerks in the face or around the eyes
- Uneven opening of the eyelids due to sagging
- "Almost stroke-like" presentation or symptoms
- Frequent or unexplained accidents, injuries, or wrecks

Cataplexy can:

- Be vague
- Occur in any muscle in the body, except for the eyes and the diaphragm
- Occur with any emotion
- Be associated with rapid recovery after only a few seconds or be delayed even up to twenty minutes, but when recovery occurs, it reverses quickly
- Cause patients to learn suppression mechanisms to avoid emotions such as pain, anger, laughter, sexual excitation, fear, and humiliation to prevent cataplexy

- Increase with poor sleep, fatigue, emotion, stress, or heavy meals
- Occur with loud noise or extreme temperature
- Cause isolation and emotional distancing

Narcolepsy can be diagnosed in two separate ways. The first is by using *The International Classification of Sleep Disorders* (ICSD-3-TR) (Medicine, 2023) in which the patient must have daily periods of irrepressible need to sleep or lapses into sleep for at least three months and other diagnostic findings using a combination of two different sleep studies, a PSG (polysomnography) or overnight sleep study, followed by an MSLT (multiple sleep latency test) or the daytime nap study. Specifically, the MSLT must demonstrate that the patient quickly goes into REM early and falls asleep quickly. Alternatively, the cerebrospinal fluid showing decreased hypocretin-1 concentration values aids in the diagnosis.

The second method involves using the Diagnostic and Statistical Manual of Mental Disorders 5th Edition (DSM-V), the American Psychiatric Association's professional reference book on mental health and brain-related conditions (Association, 2013).

The DSM-V criteria state that a patient must have an irrepressible need to sleep, lapses into sleep, or napping occurring within the same day at least three times per week over three months and at least **ONE** of the following:

- Cataplexy
- A hypocretin deficiency
- PSG and MSLT findings, which are diagnostic of narcolepsy (the PSG/MSLT is not absolutely required for DSM-V diagnosis, unlike the ICSD-3 criteria)

**One negative MSLT does not exclude the diagnosis of narcolepsy, and it may need to be repeated.

Certain medications and medical conditions can affect the test results.

Additionally, an MSLT is not required if the other DSM-5 criteria are met.

Treatment of narcolepsy:

The treatment of narcolepsy is multifactorial and must include a behavioral component, including maintaining a regular sleep schedule, scheduling daily naps, exercising, seeking education about the illness, sharing information with family members and friends, and, if necessary, work or academic accommodations. Online support groups such as those offered at Wake Up Narcolepsy, the Narcolepsy Network, Project Sleep, the Sleep Foundation, the Hypersomnia Foundation, etc., are incredibly valuable to patients and their families.

Medications used to treat narcolepsy include:

- The Oxybates: Xywav/Xyrem/Lumryz
  - Sodium oxybate (Xyrem) was one of the first unique treatments for narcolepsy, treating both excessive daytime sleepiness and cataplexy. Xyrem is given once at bedtime and repeated once at night about four hours later. A once-nightly version of sodium oxybate has been released and is called Lumryz.
  - Xywav is the second generation of Xyrem and is a low-sodium version, which may be cardioprotective and reduce the risk of other physical health disorders so commonly found with narcolepsy.

- ○ While taken at night, these medications build up and provide both day and nighttime improvement in symptoms of both sleepiness and cataplexy.

- Wakix (pitolisant)
  - ○ Wakix is FDA-approved for the treatment of both excessive daytime sleepiness and cataplexy in narcolepsy. It is not a controlled substance, which is an advantage over many of the other therapies used for narcolepsy, leading to increased ease of use. It can be taken once each day in the morning and may be used in combination with other narcolepsy treatments if necessary.

- Wake-promoting agents/stimulants

  Somnolytics are used to decrease daytime sedation and increase alertness. These substances help with sleepiness but do not treat cataplexy if present.

  Examples include:
  - ○ Provigil (modafinil) and Nuvigil (armodafinil)
  - ○ Sunosi (solriamfetol) is FDA-approved for both the sleepiness of narcolepsy and the residual sleepiness of OSA.
  - ○ Stimulants are used to increase alertness, and there are some advantages to offering long-acting and short-acting versions to help control symptoms throughout the day. A short-acting medication used as needed is frequently provided for days of severe excessive sleepiness or prolonged need for wakefulness. The shorter-acting versions are also used PRN when driving or in other situations where safety may be an issue.

○ Stimulants include such medications as Ritalin or Concerta (methylphenidate), Adderall (dextroamphetamine/amphetamine), Focalin (dexmethylphenidate), Zenzedi (dextroamphetamine sulfate), or Dexedrine (dextroamphetamine).

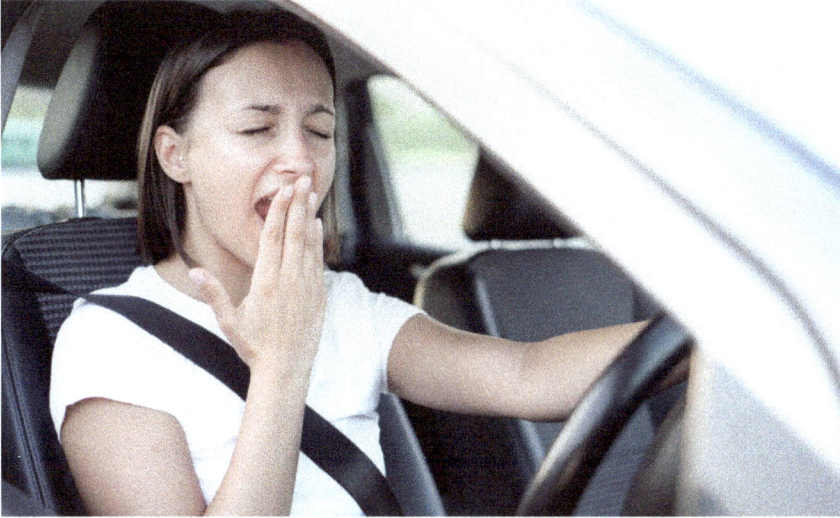

- Antidepressants
  ○ Antidepressants such as SSRI antidepressants and Tricyclic antidepressants are REM-suppressing and may help treat cataplexy, hypnogogic hallucinations, sleep paralysis, insomnia, and any co-existing depression or possibly anxiety.

- Miscellaneous medications
  ○ Various other interventions have been reported over the years, including medications such as Strattera (atomoxetine), Emsam or Eldepryl (selegiline), Baclofen, and Sanorex or Mazanor (mazindol). New studies focusing on orexin and possibly T-cell modifying medications are being considered.

Idiopathic Hypersomnia (IH)

"I'm so tired, my tired is tired."

~ Unknown

Idiopathic Hypersomnia is a disorder of persistent, excessive daytime sleepiness and great difficulty waking up. It can be associated with a very long sleep time of ten to eleven hours or more. Despite these long sleep times, their sleep is thought to be unrefreshing. There is an almost uncontrollable desire to sleep. They take long naps that are often unrefreshing. It can be very debilitating! Dauvilliers et al. (2022) provided a review of the clinical consideration of IH in which they described the excessive daytime sleepiness of IH and its associated features of sleep inertia or "sleep drunkenness," which is difficulty transitioning from sleep to wake. Patients often need multiple alarms, support from others to help them wake up, special extra loud or vibrating alarms (these can be found online), frequent phone calls from friends or family, or other creative ways to ensure they awaken for school, work, or other important appointments. And even once they wake up, they complain of feeling "half awake and half asleep." It can take a long time for them to feel fully alert.

Upon awakening, they are slow-moving, have trouble with coordination, seem confused and less alert. This is often referred to as sleep inertia, and they have drowsiness, disorientation, and impaired motor dexterity, which can last from minutes to hours (usually only fifteen to thirty minutes).

Confusional arousals or sleep drunkenness can occur upon awakening and lead to irritability and inappropriate behaviors. Their speech may be slurred, and they may have difficulty with simple tasks such as walking or dressing. They may appear disoriented and may have amnesia for the event after being fully alert.

124

IH patients often have a "brain fog" throughout the day, which is a clouding of consciousness with difficulty paying attention, being poorly aware of surroundings, confusion, forgetfulness, and decreased ability to function.

This disorder must be differentiated from narcolepsy by the presence of a symptom of muscle weakness with emotions called cataplexy in patients with narcolepsy and the absence of specific MSLT sleep test findings or abnormal cerebrospinal fluid findings diagnostic of narcolepsy.

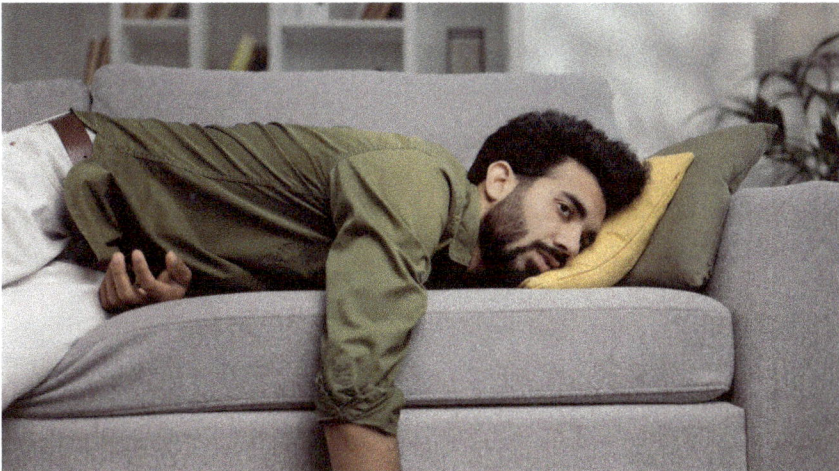

Patients with IH often have long, unrefreshing naps, as opposed to the naps in narcolepsy, which are shorter and reported as refreshing. Like narcolepsy, academic, occupational, emotional, and driving impairments can all occur. Depression and anxiety can be found in both groups as well. IH can be associated with headaches, irritability, and dizziness. If given the opportunity, they will sleep up to eleven hours or more at night, take long naps during the day, and still complain of feeling sleepy.

There is an overlap between IH and narcolepsy symptoms, and some patients previously thought to have IH are eventually diagnosed with narcolepsy after the presentation or recognition of cataplexy. Continuing to monitor for cataplexy or other symptoms of narcolepsy may lead to the need for a repeat PSG/MSLT.

Idiopathic Hypersomnia may be associated with headaches, syncope, orthostatic hypotension, and peripheral vascular complaints such as Raynaud's (a disorder in which there is decreased blood flow to the fingers and toes with stress or exposure to the cold resulting in the fingers or toes turning white or blue and eventually red when blood flow returns.) Triggers may be involved in the start of IH, such as a virus, head trauma, overexertion, anesthesia, or sudden changes to your sleep-wake schedule.

Xywav (calcium, magnesium, potassium, sodium oxybate) is the first FDA-approved treatment for IH and has significantly improved the lives of many of my patients.

Other treatments we have used off-label over the years include stimulants such as Ritalin (methylphenidate), Adderall (amphetamine/dextroamphetamine), or somnolytics such as Nuvigil (armodafinil) and Provigil (modafinil), Wellbutrin (bupropion), and other antidepressants, as well as Biaxin (clarithromycin). Wakix (pitolisant) is seeking FDA approval for this disorder.

Behavioral interventions for IH include exercise, sunlight or light therapy, avoiding alcohol and caffeine, educating family members, teachers, and employers, taking timed naps, maintaining a consistent sleep schedule, avoiding caffeine late in the day, cognitive behavioral therapy, and avoiding alcohol close to bedtime. Support groups are also available online.

Periodic Limb Movement Disorder (PLMD)

Periodic limb movement disorder is diagnosed with a PSG sleep study. A repetitive twitch or movement of the limbs during sleep causes arousal to a lighter stage of sleep or even wakefulness, leading to non-refreshing and non-restorative sleep. The movements can be mild, undetected to the eye, or more extreme. It may involve the big toe, ankle, leg, knee, hip, and upper extremities. How often it occurs during the night determines the degree of sleep disruption. Usually, patients complain of daytime fatigue, sleepiness, or even insomnia due to frequent sleep disruptions. They may be unaware they even have these movements. Sometimes, bed partners are the ones who report the movement, emphasizing the need for third-party history when evaluating sleep disorders.

It is very often associated with restless legs syndrome and is often associated with other sleep disorders such as OSA, narcolepsy, and REM behavior disorder.

It can be caused by various medications such as SSRI and SNRI antidepressants such as Effexor (venlafaxine), Cymbalta (duloxetine), Zoloft (sertraline), Prozac (fluoxetine), Elavil (amitriptyline), and Remeron (mirtazapine), as well as antihistamines such as Benadryl (diphenhydramine), antipsychotics, and Reglan (metoclopramide) which may increase PLMD.

It can run in families, be associated with anemia or diabetes, be related to smoking or obesity, and be increased by alcohol. It has been associated with B12 deficiency, low magnesium, folate deficiency, renal failure, and withdrawal of CNS depressants/sedatives/hypnotics.

Pharmacologic interventions that may be helpful include Requip (ropinirole), Mirapex (pramipexole), Sinemet (levodopa/carbidopa), Symmetrel (amantadine), opioids, Klonopin (clonazepam), Depakote (valproate), Neurontin (gabapentin), Lyrica (pregabalin), and the muscle relaxer Baclofen. Patients should be encouraged to take a multivitamin with iron. Magnesium supplementation is also beneficial. Melatonin has been found to improve some patients' periodic limb movements and arousals.

Restless Legs Syndrome (RLS)

Restless legs syndrome (Willis-Ekbom Disease) is a disorder in which patients complain of an uncomfortable sensation in their legs or arms with the desire to move, stretch, or rub these muscles. It can occur during the day or night. It usually occurs in the evening or after dinner, with increased symptoms at night. It is strongly associated with periodic limb movement disorder. It has been described as a crawling, aching, under-the-skin tingling, throbbing, itching, burning, like an electrical current, like worms or bugs crawling under the skin, or a restless feeling associated with the overwhelming desire to move, rub, or scratch the legs. It can be painful. At bedtime, patients have difficulty getting settled in or sleeping comfortably. RLS can occur in children and adults and may be especially prevalent in the elderly with multiple physical disorders. In children, it is often dismissed as "growing pains," but it may improve with a multivitamin with iron.

Movement and rubbing the legs can provide some relief. Patients may get up, walk, stretch, or "jiggle" their legs. Their covers are often messed up, and bed partners may complain about their inability to stay still. PLMD is associated with insomnia and difficulty maintaining sleep, resulting in fatigue, sleepiness complaints, and irritability or mood changes. If aroused by PLMD, the RLS cycle may start during the night.

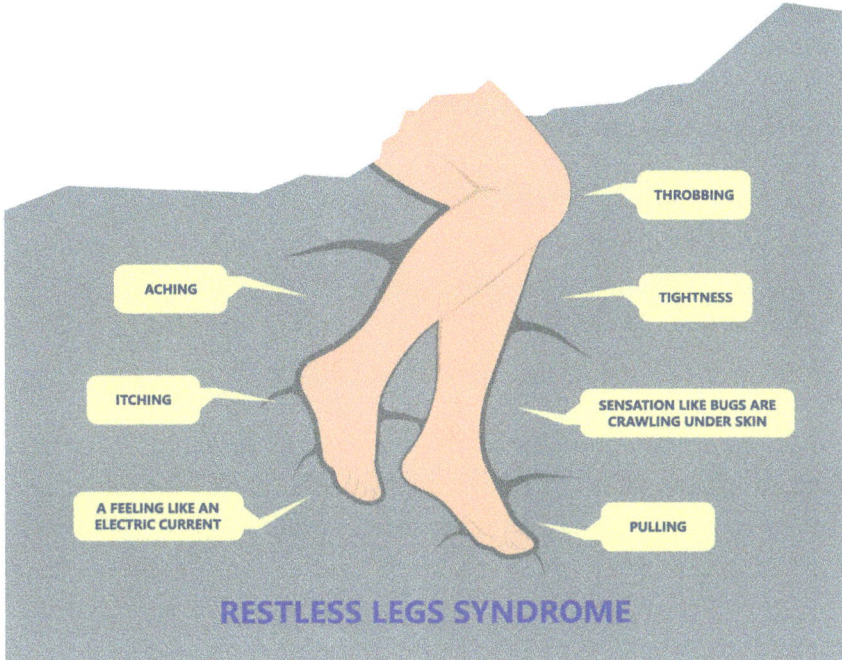

THROBBING

ACHING

TIGHTNESS

ITCHING

SENSATION LIKE BUGS ARE CRAWLING UNDER SKIN

A FEELING LIKE AN ELECTRIC CURRENT

PULLING

RESTLESS LEGS SYNDROME

RLS can be genetic and can run in families. Sleep deprivation may increase RLS. It has also been associated with medical disorders such as anemia, diabetic neuropathy, Parkinson's disease, peripheral neuropathy, uremia, chronic kidney disease, rheumatoid arthritis, gastric surgeries, pregnancy, venous insufficiency, fibromyalgia, low testosterone, MS, ADHD, and tic disorders. Stress can increase RLS, and alcohol use can contribute.

Laboratory evaluation is recommended to rule out any reversible causes. Labs should include iron, ferritin, transferrin saturation, total iron binding capacity, potassium, folate, vitamin B-12, magnesium, blood urea nitrogen, creatinine, fasting blood glucose, and thyroid stimulating hormone (TSH).

Certain medications may contribute to RLS symptoms, such as antidepressants, antipsychotics, antinausea medications, lithium, beta-blockers, and antihistamines (such as Benadryl or diphen-hydramine). Caffeine may also increase RLS.

Iron deficiency may be a significant contributor. Patients with RLS reliably respond to iron therapy if their pretreatment serum ferritin levels are less than forty-five. Vitamin and mineral supplements, including vitamin B12, vitamin C, vitamin E, and calcium, have been reported to help alleviate symptoms. Folic acid supplementation improves RLS. Magnesium supplementation is also beneficial; magnesium oil rubbed on the legs is often helpful.

Behavioral treatment include applying counter stimuli such as socks, light stretching, hot baths/showers, heating pads, and ice packs. Tasks requiring a lot of concentration at night, such as crossword puzzles, needlework, word search puzzles, computer games, etc., may decrease RLS.

Requip (ropinirole), Mirapex (pramipexole), and the Neupro patch (rotigotine) have been approved for RLS. The Neupro patch is beneficial for those with day and nighttime symptoms. Other pharmacologic interventions include dopaminergic agents such as Sinemet (carbidopa and levodopa), Parlodel (bromocriptine), or Amantadine. Other pharmacological interventions that have been used include Lyrica (pregabalin), opioids, Klonopin (clonazepam), Neurontin (gabapentin), or Clonidine. TENS units (transcutaneous electrical nerve stimulation) can reduce RLS symptoms. A hot bath with Epsom Salts may also provide some relief.

Nocturnal Leg Cramps

Leg cramps, or "Charley horses," are sudden, involuntary muscle spasms that cause intense pain. They usually occur in the calf but may also occur in the foot or thigh.

The exact cause is unknown, but they may be associated with muscle fatigue or overwork, electrolyte deficiency such as potassium, calcium, or magnesium, or due to certain medications such as diuretics or statin medications. They can be related to nerve disorders or peripheral vascular disease. Excessive running, standing on the legs, walking up inclines, etc., may also contribute. Medications that have been associated with leg cramps include antidepressants such as Prozac (fluoxetine) and Zoloft (Sertraline), the statin drugs used to lower cholesterol, diuretics such as Lasix (furosemide) or hydrochlorothiazide, Premarin (estrogen), Ambien (zolpidem), Neurontin (gabapentin) or Lyrica (Pregabalin). There are many others, too. You may want to ask your pharmacist to see if any of the medications you are taking could be contributing if they become chronic.

They can occur during pregnancy, with thyroid disorders, in Parkinson's, in chronic kidney disease, with alcohol use, and with dehydration.

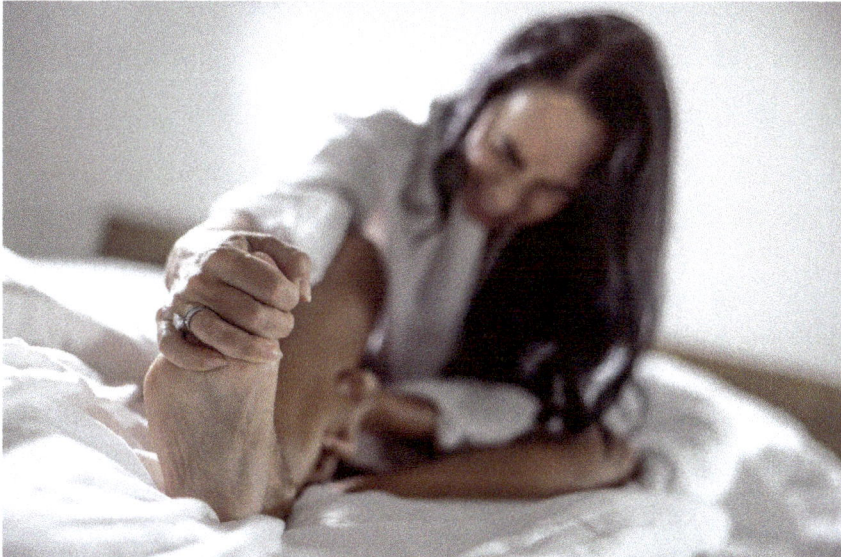

Treatments include stretching, massage, magnesium oil or spray to rub on the muscle, applying heat or ice, Quinine or Tonic Water, vitamin E, Verapamil, or Neurontin (gabapentin). Additionally, potassium, magnesium, vitamin B complex, and calcium supplementation may be of benefit. As has heel walking, pickle juice has also been reported to be helpful. The muscle rub-on creams such as Icy Hot®, Biofreeze®, Bengay®, Voltaren® (diclofenac) Topical, Asper cream®, Capsaicin cream, Tiger Balm®, Blue-Emu®, and others have all been reported by my patients to provide some relief.

If leg cramps frequently recur, taking magnesium glycinate every evening may help, or possibly other medications. One might also consider their shoes and other things that could strain the muscles throughout the day. Drinking plenty of fluids daily, avoiding dehydration, and trying light stretching each evening before bedtime may also help. Hot baths with Epsom salts are another option. If severe and/or recurring, a medical evaluation with labs may be indicated.

Nocturia

Nocturia is the name for getting up to go to the bathroom at night. If this occurs infrequently, it is usually not an issue. It can be very disruptive for those who have to get up to go to the toilet almost nightly and multiple times during the night. It can lead to fragmented, non-restorative sleep by waking frequently and returning to the lighter stages of sleep. Without uninterrupted sleep, your body does not have time to cycle into the deeper stages of sleep. Nocturia can also be associated with nighttime falls, as patients may not be fully awake or cannot see well in dimly lit areas with only a night light.

Many issues can cause nocturia. One of the most common is drinking excessive fluids in the evening and before bedtime—also fluids associated with urinary frequency, such as caffeine and alcohol. Even carbonated drinks, acidic juices (orange juice and grapefruit), and sparking water can irritate the bladder, causing increased urination, as can artificial sweeteners.

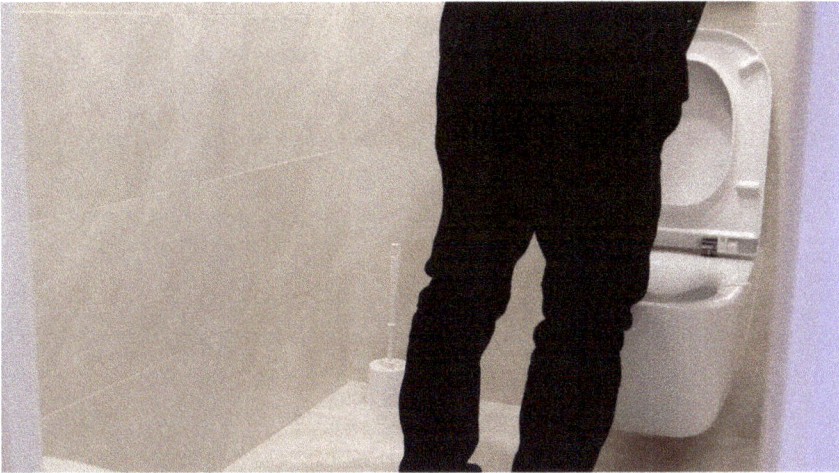

Prostate enlargement in men is a frequent cause of nocturia.

Hormonal Issues, such as a decline in estrogen with menopause and low testosterone in men, may contribute. Treatment with hormone replacement therapy and testosterone supplementation may be beneficial. Diabetes is another cause of frequent urination at night.

Sleep apnea can lead to increased urine production and may also be associated with nocturia.

Other medical disorders such as hypertension, cardiovascular disorders, heart failure, or kidney failure and their treatments can result in frequent bathroom trips at night.

Medications with a diuretic such as Lasix (furosemide), HCTZ (hydrochlorothiazide), and Aldactone (spironolactone) can increase urination. Other medications also have a side effect of nocturia, such as blood pressure medications including beta-blockers, calcium channel blockers, ACE inhibitors, and angiotensin receptor blockers, as well as psychotropics such as lithium, antipsychotics (for example, Abilify (aripiprazole), Risperdal (risperidone), Zyprexa (olanzapine), Mellaril (thioridazine), Clozaril (clozapine), as well as some antidepressants including some SSRIs, SNRIs, and TCAs. Sodium glucose co-transporter-2 inhibitors (SGLT2) like Jardiance (empagliflozin), Farxiga (dapagliflozin), and Invokana (canagliflozin) can also contribute. Even benzodiazepines such as Xanax (alprazolam), Ativan (lorazepam), and Valium (diazepam) can cause frequent urination.

High calcium levels, a small or overactive bladder, and urinary tract infections can increase urinary frequency and nocturia.

Not completely emptying the bladder can lead to repeated bathroom trips. Helpful hints here include paying attention, leaning slightly forward, and trying to urinate again while you are still sitting there.

Pelvic organ prolapse, restless legs syndrome, edema, and obesity are other associated disorders found with nocturia.

Tips for dealing with nocturia include:

- Go to the bathroom immediately before sleep.
- Restrict fluids in the evenings.
- Avoid alcohol and caffeine in the evenings, as this can increase urination.
- Talk with your doctor and pharmacist to evaluate what medications you are taking in the evening and at bedtime to see if any of those may contribute. Many different drugs can cause increased urinary frequency or nocturia as a potential side effect.

- Take an afternoon nap to allow your body to absorb fluids.
- Pelvic floor therapy can strengthen pelvic floor muscles and be helpful.
- Wear compression stockings.
- A few of the meds that are helpful treatment interventions include Myrbetriq (Mirabegron), Enablex (Darifenacin), Ditropan (oxybutynin), Detrol (tolterodine), and DDAVP (desmopressin).

Enuresis

Bedwetting or urinary incontinence is called enuresis and is involuntary, unintentional urinating at night during sleep. Enuresis is more commonly seen in children but can occur in adults, especially with certain medications and medical issues such as obstructive sleep apnea, alcohol use, sleepwalking, diabetes, seizures, urinary tract infections, an overactive bladder, and many other problems. Multiple medications may contribute to enuresis, and sometimes, it may be as easy as switching your medications to AM or afternoon dosing after discussing this with your provider and/or pharmacist.

Pharmacologic treatments include DDAVP (desmopressin), Ditropan (oxybutynin), Tofranil (Imipramine), and other agents.

There is a treatment called alarm therapy for children, a system attached to the child's underwear that alarms with the first wetness detection. With time, it can train the brain to wake up before getting wet. Pelvic floor therapy, biofeedback, avoiding evening and bedtime drinks, urinating just before bed, and urotherapy (which involves education, behavioral modifications, and support to improve bladder function, thereby teaching children to use the bathroom regularly) are all helpful behavioral interventions.

Nocturnal Gastroesophageal Reflux

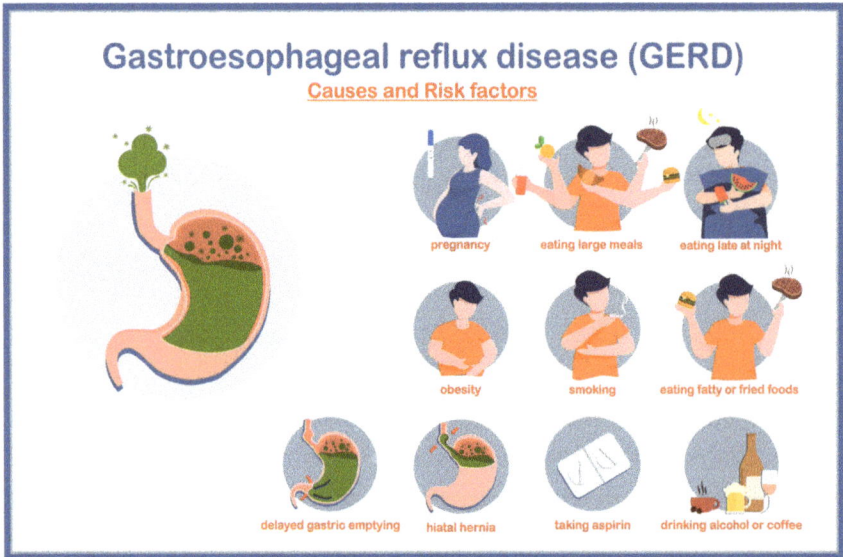

Gastroesophageal reflux disease (GERD)
Causes and Risk factors

pregnancy — eating large meals — eating late at night
obesity — smoking — eating fatty or fried foods
delayed gastric emptying — hiatal hernia — taking aspirin — drinking alcohol or coffee

Gastroesophageal reflux can cause heartburn, chest pain, sore throat, and even voice changes. These symptoms can occur at any time of the day, but they can be incredibly disruptive at night, interfering with sleep quantity and quality.

Behavioral interventions are helpful and include things such as elevating the head of the bed, sleeping on the left side, sleeping on a triangle wedge pillow, avoiding large meals or excessive fluids close to bedtime, reducing alcohol intake in the evening and before bedtime, stopping smoking, weight management, and identifying meals or beverages most likely to cause reflux. Spicy foods, high-sugar foods/drinks, caffeine, dairy, acidic foods and drinks (such as citrus fruits and juices, tomato-based foods and tomato juice, or vinegar), carbonated beverages, chocolate, and fatty foods may all contribute. Even peppermint can increase GERD.

Medications used to treat GERD include:

- Antacids
- H2 blockers like Tagamet (cimetidine) or Pepcid (famotidine) can increase slow-wave sleep and improve sleep quality
- Proton pump inhibitors such as Prilosec (omeprazole), Nexium (esomeprazole), and Protonix (pantoprazole)
- Prokinetic agents like Reglan (metoclopramide)

GERD and obstructive sleep apnea are bidirectional, meaning they each can make the other worse. Apnea can increase pressure and decrease intrathoracic pressure, leading to GERD. GERD can block the airway and increase apnea. Aggressive treatment of both can help the other if both disorders are present.

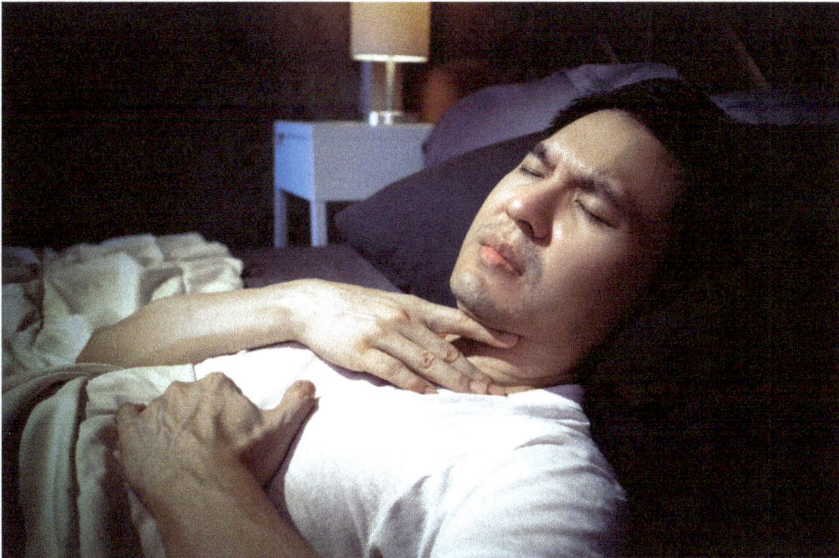

Nightmares

Nightmares are usually REM-related symptoms that may be so severe that people are afraid to go to sleep at night or to take naps during the day. The degree of detail my patients tell me is scary just to hear about during the daytime, let alone experience at night. Nightmares can be precipitated by stress, sleep deprivation, various medications, sleep disorders, irregular sleep schedules, watching or witnessing aggressive content, trauma associated with PTSD, borderline personality disorder, and even brought on by the foods you eat. Some have suggested that eating spicy or heavy meals before bedtime can induce nightmares. Sleep disorders associated with nightmares include narcolepsy, sleep apnea, irregular sleep-wake schedules, insomnia, and REM sleep behavior disorder. It has been reported that sleeping in a room that is too hot or too cold can also lead to nightmares.

Treatment of nightmares includes:

- Medications such as Minipress (prazosin), Halcion (triazolam), Zyprexa (olanzapine), Risperdal (risperidone), Abilify (aripiprazole), Catapress (clonidine), Periactin (cyproheptadine), Neurontin (gabapentin), Luvox (fluvoxamine), Topamax (topiramate), Desyrel (trazodone), and tricyclic Antidepressants (Morgenthaler et al., 2018).
- Consider environmental issues, such as sleeping in a cooler room to decrease the risk of nightmares.
- Limit caffeine, alcohol, and nicotine.
- Avoid spicy, sugary, or heavy meals before bedtime.
- Limit exposure to the news, scary movies, gruesome books, murder shows, or thinking of past abuse before sleep.
- Cognitive behavioral therapy for nightmares includes:
  - *Imagery rehearsal therapy (IRT)* is a form of cognitive behavior therapy that involves thinking about the

dream, writing it down, and consciously rewriting it with a positive or neutral ending. After changing the dream story to a less distressing or positive outcome, patients are advised to mentally rehearse the dream for 10–20 minutes daily, paying attention to all five senses and practicing relaxation instead of alarming sensations. They are advised to try this for at least two weeks. The goal of IRT is to desensitize the patient to the fear of a nightmare and increase a sense of control over nightmares.

A fascinating podcast by Barry Krakow, MD, can be found on *The Carlat Psychiatry Podcast* called "Why Nightmares Matter," in which he suggested asking patients if they thought about their dreams during the day, evaluating for sleep apnea, as well as practicing the revised versions of the nightmares daily. (For more information, visit www. barrykrakowmd.com.) Lancee, Effting, and Kunze (Lancee et al., 2021) published an article using telephone- guided IRT for nightmares and found decreased frequency, decreased distress, and decreased severity of nightmares.

- ○ *Exposure, relaxation, and rescripting therapy or ERRT* (Davis & Wright, 2006) involves psychoeducation about nightmares, relaxation training, sleep hygiene, and nightmare exposure and rescripting. Patients are gradually exposed to the content of the nightmare in a safe environment, along with relaxation techniques such as deep breathing and progressive muscle relaxation. They are helped to rewrite the dream content more neutrally.
- ○ *Lucid dreaming therapy (LDT)* is a psychotherapeutic approach involving cognitive restructuring in which the patient is aware that they are dreaming and

seeks to reduce nightmares by increasing control over the content of dreams, developing insight into personal emotions, thoughts, and behaviors surrounding the dream content, and working on developing problem-solving skills (Holzinger et al., 2020). Holzinger et al. report, "Lucid dreaming (LD) is a learnable and effective strategy to cope with nightmares and positively affects other sleep variables."

Stephen LaBerge, a psychophysiologist and leader in research from Stanford University with his continued research at "The Lucidity Institute" wrote a book in 2009 entitled "Lucid Dreaming: A Concise Guide to Awakening in Your Dreams and in Your Life" (LaBerge, 2009). Many books on this subject have been written over the years incorporating the general techniques described below.

LDT includes:

- ✦ Reality Checks
- ✦ Dream Journaling
- ✦ The Wake Back to Bed Technique (WBTB) which involves setting the alarm five to six hours after going to sleep, staying awake for 20–30 minutes, focusing on lucid dreaming, and going back to sleep while thinking of the dream. This technique is believed to wake the patient during REM sleep (LaBerge, S., Phillips, L., & Levita, 1994) (Shredl, 2020).
- ✦ Mnemonic Induction of Lucid Dreams (MILD) is a technique in which patients try to recognize they are dreaming and make statements like "the next time I dream, I will remember I am dreaming" (La Berge, 1980).

> ✦ Meditation & Relaxation during the day can be helpful and is also used if one awakens from a nightmare.
> ✦ The Sleep Foundation website has an interesting article entitled "How to Lucid Dream: Expert Tips and Tricks" (Bryan and Singh 2024) that you may want to review.

- Progressive muscle relaxation, as previously mentioned, can also be of benefit.
- Sleep hygiene—Sleep deprivation can cause REM rebound sleep, increasing dreaming and the potential for nightmares. Maintaining a regular sleep schedule can promote healthy sleeping and decrease the risk of nightmares.
- Look for any triggers to nightmares when they do occur to help decrease their frequency in the future.
- Keep a journal for dream analysis.

Night Terrors or Sleep Terrors

Night terrors are sudden awakenings with intense fear, confusion, increased heart rate, sweating, sometimes screaming or yelling out, panic-like symptoms, even crying out, and possibly kicking, thrashing about, or hitting. These episodes are alarming to those around the person having a night terror. They are more common in children and may be associated with sleepwalking. Most children will outgrow these episodes. They are often brief but can last much longer and are associated with stage 3 NREM sleep. Adults with night terrors frequently have a coexisting history of anxiety disorders, PTSD, depression, and possibly personality disorders. They can be associated with other sleep disorders such as sleep apnea, restless legs syndrome, and periodic limb movement disorder. Low blood sugar levels have been associated with some pediatric and adult cases. They can run in families, increase with stress and fever, and increase after sleep deprivation. A full bladder can also be a precipitating factor, so emptying the bladder immediately before going to bed and restricting fluids for an hour or two before sleep may be helpful. Alcohol and caffeine can increase night terrors and should be decreased or avoided in those having frequent episodes. Usually, the person having the night terror does not remember the content and goes back to sleep.

If night terrors are recurring and/or severe, treatment options include sleep hygiene, reassurance, education about precipitating factors, environmental safety, hypnosis, cognitive behavioral therapy, and, if very significant, antidepressants or benzodiazepines (such as Klonopin). If there is a pattern in which the night terrors occur at a particular time of the night, anticipatory awakening or arousing about thirty minutes to one hour before that time can help prevent them.

REM Behavior Disorder (RBD)

REM behavior disorder occurs when there is an "unhooking" of the paralysis usually associated with REM sleep, allowing patients to act out their dreams in a dramatic or occasionally violent manner. Depending on the dream content, this can involve vocalizations, physical movements, or even violent movements. It may occur in both the pediatric and adult population but is more common in men over fifty years of age, in those with PTSD, when withdrawing from alcohol or sedatives, and there is an increased risk in those with Parkinson's disease or Lewy body dementia. It can also increase in times of stress.

Some medications can be associated with RBD, such as antidepressants, Alzheimer's treatments, Remeron (mirtazapine), Barbiturates, Eldepryl (selegiline), and Meprobamate.

Treatment of REM behavior disorder involves removing any situations or medications that may precipitate symptoms like those listed previously. If needed, medicines that have been used include Klonopin (clonazepam), Xanax (alprazolam), Tegretol (carbamazepine), Clonidine, L-dopa, melatonin, Mirapex (pramipexole), and Paxil (paroxetine.) Klonopin is the most commonly recommended treatment. Another treatment option is the Exelon patch (transdermal rivastigmine) where RBD is associated with mild cognitive impairment (Howell et al., 2023).

The patients and their families should be made aware of this disorder, and arrangements should be made for a safe sleeping environment if actions are more violent.

I have had one sweet little lady in whom we diagnosed this disorder after the death of her husband. She moved in with one of her sons, and they brought her to me for an evaluation, thinking she may be psychotic or something because she was yelling out, singing, and making significant movements nightly in her sleep. When we studied her in the sleep lab, she sang religious songs during REM sleep and made movements as if cooking breakfast. A little therapy and a sprinkle of Klonopin alleviated her symptoms.

Others have been more aggressive, with one patient punching his wife in his sleep after being happily and peacefully married for many years. He was dreaming he was in a bar fight. RBD is associated with other neurodegenerative disorders such as Parkinson's disease, multisystem atrophy, and Lewy body dementia. We felt his RBD was associated with his onset of Parkinson's.

There has been some suggestion that a history of a head injury, smoking, farming, or exposure to occupational pesticides may be linked to this disorder.

I have had patients dive out a window, one who kneed his wife during their sleep, and another broke a coffee table, but these are unusual cases. Most are less severe and respond well to medications. Some must sleep in another room without a lot of furniture. There are extreme cases, but those are far less common.

Sexsomnia

Sexsomnia is engaging in any form of sexual activity during sleep, including intercourse, masturbation, fondling, making sexual noises or movements, or even aggressive or inappropriate behavior without full awareness or even memory of the event. Sexsomnia is a type of NREM parasomnia of sleep and can be associated with other sleep disorders, anxiety, depression, substance abuse, seizures, and sleep deprivation. Cases have been reported with some medications, like over-the-counter sleep aids. It can also be associated with sleepwalking or sleep-talking.

Treatment recommendations include identifying and treating other contributing disorders and, if necessary, Klonopin (clonazepam). Behavioral interventions involve avoiding sleep deprivation, avoiding alcohol, sleeping in a separate room if required, avoiding sleeping around strangers or minors, and psychotherapy.

Hypnic Jerks

Hypnic jerks or "sleep starts" are involuntary, brief muscle jerks or twitching occurring with the onset of sleep involving the arms or legs and associated with a sense of falling, a dream at the onset of sleep, a startle, or a sensory flash. Triggers include sleep deprivation, other sleep disorders such as apnea, emotional stress, caffeine, nicotine, intense fatigue, physical exercise, or periods of increased stress. They are benign and may occur in up to 70% of the population at some point in their life.

Exploding Head Syndrome

Exploding head syndrome is another disorder that occurs with the transition into sleep and is associated with an abrupt awakening with the sensation of a bursting in the head, explosion, thunderclap, crashing sound, or even the sound of a gunshot. It is alarming, confusing, and oftentimes frightening to the patient. A review by Khan and Slowik in *StatPearls* (2025) reported that treatment usually includes education and reassurance, anxiety treatment, treatment of cooccurring sleep disorders, stress management, and sleep hygiene. If necessary, case reports have demonstrated improvement with Klonopin (clonazepam), Trileptal (Oxcarbazepine), Anafranil (clomipramine), Elavil (amitriptyline), Topamax (topiramate), Cymbalta (duloxetine), and Procardia (nifedipine). Other medications have also been used in isolated case reports.

Sleep Paralysis

Sleep paralysis occurs during the transition from sleep to waking, and the patient briefly feels awake but cannot move or speak. This is believed to be due to waking during REM sleep, with the muscle paralysis of REM sleep continuing. It is usually brief but can last for several minutes and may provoke anxiety, especially until the diagnosis is made and the patient is educated about the disorder and what factors may precipitate it. Isolated events occur in about 30% of the population during their lifetime and are usually associated with sleep deprivation. Sleep paralysis may be part of the symptoms present with narcolepsy. There is another form called recurrent isolated sleep paralysis that occurs in the absence of narcolepsy.

There is a familial form that runs in families. Sleep deprivation, irregular sleep-wake schedules, shift work, alcohol use, insufficient sleep syndrome (a disorder of persistent lack of adequate sleep leading to impaired functioning, irritability, decreased concentration/attention, poor motivation, and excessive fatigue or sleepiness), anxiolytic medication use, and sleeping in the supine position are possible triggers. It has been associated with obstructive sleep apnea, exploding head syndrome, nocturnal leg cramps, idiopathic hypersomnia, bipolar disorder, hypertension, and Wilson's disease. Sometimes, these events are mislabeled as nocturnal panic attacks.

These events usually resolve spontaneously, but being touched or spoken to or making intense efforts to move can help end the situation. Suggested treatments during the episode include moving your eyes back and forth from right to left, blinking, or focusing on moving one finger or slight body movement. Trying to make a noise, distract yourself, force an intense movement such as coughing or jerking, and focus on deep breathing have also been helpful. Avoiding sleep deprivation and avoiding sleeping in the supine position have also been suggested to decrease the risk of sleep paralysis.

Sleepwalking (Somnambulism)

Sleepwalking involves getting out of bed as if awake while sleeping. During that time, the patient may engage in dream acting behavior, routine activities, or complex behavior such as leaving the house and driving. Behaviors can be simple, complex, protracted, goal-directed, or even sexual in nature.

The episode often begins as a confusional arousal, and the sleepwalking becomes an extension of the episode. Confusional arousals occur when the patient is in bed; if the patient leaves the bed, sleepwalking has started.

They may appear awake but usually do not remember events during or after the event.

It can run in families and can be associated with sleep deprivation, irregular sleep schedules, drinking too much alcohol, stress, anxiety, having a full bladder, being startled by a noise, or being touched. It can increase with certain medications or be associated with hyperthyroidism, Parkinson's, asthma, other sleep disorders such as sleep apnea, mental health issues such as PTSD, anxiety, or depression, or with seizures. A fever can also precipitate it. Certain medications may trigger sleepwalking, such as Ambien (zolpidem), Seroquel (quetiapine), or Lopressor (metoprolol). It is associated with NREM sleep and is more common in children. It usually occurs in the first two or three hours of falling asleep. It may increase when sleeping in a strange environment.

To help those with sleepwalking, make a loud noise, or start a conversation from a safe distance. If you touch them or get too close, they may lash out verbally or physically. Try to guide them back to bed gently.

Environmental safety should be considered for frequent sleepwalking, such as door alarms, safety gates at the top of stairs, locking up car keys or weapons, and keeping doors and windows locked.

I once had a patient with severe sleepwalking who left the house one night, drove his car, bought beer at the local gas station (he was not an alcohol drinker), parked the car in the front yard, sat the beer on the coffee table without opening it, went back to bed, and was utterly confused when confronted by his wife the following day. His sleepwalking became so severe that she had to hide the car keys each night in different locations (often in the freezer in a container). We discovered it was a medication change that precipitated sleepwalking.

Kids are especially prone to sleepwalking in a new environment, when stressed, sleep deprived, or when running a fever. I had one little girl who would get up sleepwalking, leave the house, and be out front swinging under the big tree in the middle of the night. This was terrifying for her parents! We put an ankle bracelet with jingle bells around her ankles, had door alarms in the house, installed a very high lock on the front door that she could not reach, and her parents moved their bedroom closer to her room.

People who sleepwalk may use the bathroom in unusual places (like the closet), consume unusual foods, or even cook in the kitchen. They may find food remnants in their bed, including jars of peanut butter. Sleepwalking may lead to weight gain.

Treatment usually involves removing or limiting situations that increase sleepwalking, as mentioned above, timed awakenings about thirty minutes to one hour before the usual episode of sleepwalking, aggressively looking at safety issues, improving sleep hygiene, avoiding sleep deprivation, avoiding alcohol before bedtime, treating any underlying conditions, melatonin, sedatives like benzodiazepines, CBT (cognitive behavioral therapy), and possibly a trial of calcium and magnesium. Other treatments that have been used but are not FDA-approved for this disorder include Neurontin (gabapentin), Trazodone, and Estazolam.

Nocturnal Eating

Excessive eating at night must be differentiated between:

1) Nocturnal eating disorder
2) Sleep-related eating disorder

With **nocturnal eating disorder,** the patient consumes more than 25–50% of their calories between 8 PM and 6 AM. There is a complete preservation of consciousness.

Nocturnal eating disorder has been associated with precipitation factors such as sleep deprivation or disruptions of sleep by GERD, and these issues should be addressed. Reports have also linked abnormalities in melatonin and leptin as being involved. Often, this is a learned behavior, and some behavioral interventions may also be beneficial.

Treatment options for this disorder are behavioral interventions, morning light therapy, relaxation therapy, treatment of anxiety, and, if necessary, medications like Zoloft (sertraline) and Topamax (topiramate).

Other medication treatments that have been tried including Klono-pin (clonazepam), Prozac (fluoxetine), Luvox (fluvoxamine), Desyrel (trazodone), and Wellbutrin (bupropion).

Sleep-related eating disorder is a type of parasomnia involving involuntary drinking or eating during the main sleep period and even preparing food during the night with little to no recall in the morning. There is partial or complete amnesia for the eating episodes. This type of disorder is strongly associated with other sleep disorders. It is associated with consuming peculiar foods, morning anorexia, insomnia, daytime fatigue, and occasionally self-injurious behaviors because of the dangerous behaviors in pursuit of food/drink. It can be associated with the use of medications such as Ambien (zolpidem), Restoril (temazepam), Elavil (amitriptyline), Zyprexa (olanzapine), Risperdal (risperidone), and other antipsychotics. Treatment of this disorder is often successful with dopamine agonist medications such as Requip (ropinirole), Mirapex (pramipexole), Sinemet (carbidopa/levodopa), Parlodel (bromocriptine), or Amantadine (symmetrel). It can be associated with periodic limb movement disorder, sleepwalking, or other parasomnias. It can be dangerous if someone is cooking, using a knife, opening cans, etc.

Bruxism

Bruxism is repeatedly grinding or crunching of the teeth during sleep, often associated with increased stress levels. Symptoms can occur in the daytime as well. It is often associated with pre-existing dental, mandibular, or maxillary conditions, such as dental disease or malocclusion. In fact, a dentist may be the first to recognize this disorder. It can result in headaches, tooth pain, chipped teeth, jaw pain, and noise that disrupts bed partners. In addition to stress, other contributing factors include excessive caffeine use, alcohol, smoking, and certain medications such as stimulants and SSRI antidepressants. Evaluation should consist of a dental examination. Patients may require a rubber mouth guard over their teeth to prevent further dental or jaw damage.

B R U X I S M

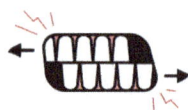

GRINDING

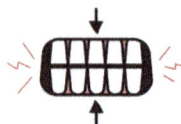

CLENCHING

Deficiencies in magnesium, calcium, and both vitamin D and B have been reported. Stress reduction techniques using relaxation training, biofeedback, or psychotherapy may be beneficial. Magnesium supplementation, muscle relaxers, Botox, anticonvulsants such as gabapentin, dopamine agonists such as levodopa and bromocriptine, benzodiazepines such as clonazepam, antidepressants such as amitriptyline, and antihistamines such as hydroxyzine, as well as removing any medications that could be contributing, are medication treatments. If sleep apnea is present, treatment of the apnea may help to relieve bruxism. Kuang et al. reported an increased association with bruxism and GERD, obstructive sleep apnea, sleep-related epilepsy, restless legs syndrome, periodic limb movement disorder, and REM behavior disorder (Kuang et al., 2022).

Confusional Arousals (Elpenor Syndrome)

Confusional arousals are thought to be an NREM parasomnia associated with an abnormal sleep-wake transition associated with difficulty awaking from sleep and during the transition being groggy, disoriented, having poor coordination, irritability, slurred or slowed speech, inappropriate or strange behavior, and afterward little recall of the episode. Injury to self or others has been reported on rare occasions. Family members are often very concerned after the confusional arousals. It can occur as part of the sleep disorder idiopathic hypersomnia or seen in other sleep disorders such as sleep apnea. They usually occur in the first couple of hours of sleep and can be precipitated by being suddenly awakened by a loud noise, an alarm, or a telephone ringing. Sleep deprivation, alcohol use, hypnotic/tranquilizer use, shift work, smoking, bipolar disorder, and other circadian rhythm sleep disorders have been associated with this disorder.

Sleep Texting

Sleep texting is not an official diagnosis; it is a parasomnia that occurs when someone messages or responds to a text message in their sleep and does not remember doing it. Like sleepwalking and those who talk in their sleep, they are unaware of their behavior. As with other parasomnias, sleep deprivation, stress, alcohol, fevers, and certain medications such as Ambien (zolpidem) may increase the risk of this behavior. If it is a recurring issue, the patient should keep their phone away from the bed, decrease the above-mentioned risk factors, and review medications or even supplements that may be contributing.

Sleep-related Groaning (Catathrenia)

Sleep-related groaning is a sleep disorder associated with loud, prolonged moaning sounds during the night with exhalation or breathing out. It differs from sleep apnea in that snoring occurs while breathing in. It is not related to respiratory pauses but can be associated with slowing the respiratory rate. It can be very alarming to bed partners or others around as they fear they may be in pain or having difficulty breathing. The noise can be monotone, sexual, humming, grunting, or squeaking.

A sleep study may be necessary to rule out other sleep disorders.

Treatments for this disorder include oral appliances, tonsil and adenoid removal, trimming or removing the uvula, and sometimes CPAP. Using a pillow with good neck support has also been suggested.

Chapter 12

Tackling Insomnia!

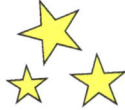

*"Whether you think you can or
you think you can't—you are right."*

~ Henry Ford

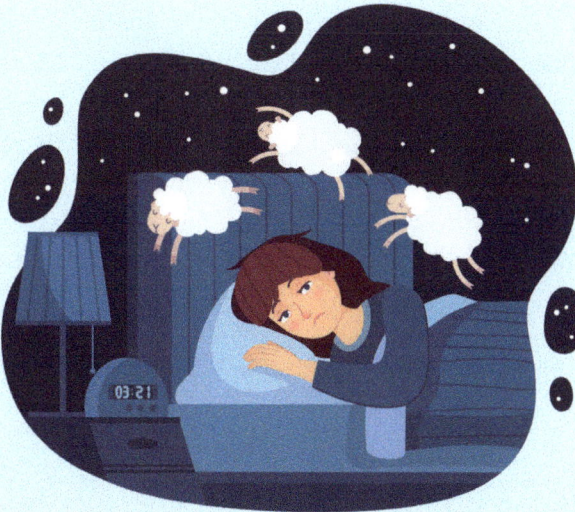

WHAT CAUSES INSOMNIA?

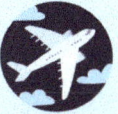 CROSSING TIME ZONES

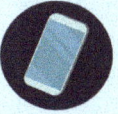 BLUE LIGHT

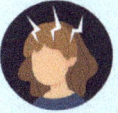 STRESS

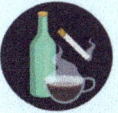 ALCOHOL, SMOKING OR CAFFEINE

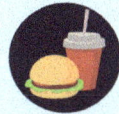 HEAVY FOOD

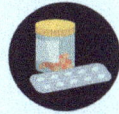 MEDICINES

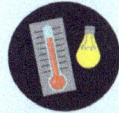 ENVIRONMENTAL FACTORS

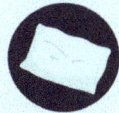 UNCOMFORTABLE BED OR PILLOW

"Tackle" seems like a big word, but for those of you who have insomnia, it can often feel like you have to gear up, put your head down, and try to "tackle" all of the issues coming at you, preventing you from sleeping each night. Instead of sleep being a peaceful, restful, restorative event, it often feels like you are on a front-line defense fighting off each of the issues, trying to prevent your overall amount of sleep and quality of sleep each night from being disturbed. Once we identify all contributing factors, the task becomes more manageable. You are more likely to sleep when you feel less overwhelmed and more optimistic about your sleep. If you focus on your insomnia and inability to sleep, you will likely have more trouble sleeping. My hope for you is that this book will help you identify ways to overcome insomnia, which often involves confidence-building strategies, practice, a different "recipe" at various times, and conscious awareness of when things are going astray.

As mentioned throughout this book and diagramed above, many contributing factors to disrupted nocturnal sleep exist.

Many sleep disorders are associated with insomnia, and there are some specific insomnia-related disorders. Medications, substance abuse, anxiety, depression, relationship stress, financial issues, physical pain, other medical disorders, poor sleep hygiene, environmental issues, and a variety of different things can contribute. We will now discuss a few more causes of insomnia before we tackle its treatment.

Psychophysiologic Insomnia

Psychophysiologic insomnia is a disorder of initiating or maintaining sleep secondary to tension and learned sleep-preventing associations. It can be due to a combination of psychological and physiological factors such as anxiety and worry about sleep, obsessive rumination, and negative thoughts. Patients with this disorder can fall asleep unintentionally but have great difficulty sleeping at night during required sleep times and with naps. It is associated with hyperarousal when trying to sleep, obsessive worries about sleep, and the consequences of their lack of sleep on their ability to function the next day. This hyperfocus on sleep can lead to obsessive ruminations about sleep during the day almost every day, which can be "paralyzing" in their ability to function, creating a vicious cycle.

Sleep State Misperception/Paradoxical Insomnia

"I dream so vividly about not being asleep that I don't think I'm sleeping when people tell me I am actually sleeping and even snoring."

~ previous patient

When the patient's interpretation of how they sleep does not match up with the findings on the overnight PSG sleep study examination, we have what is called sleep state misperception or what is sometimes referred to as paradoxical insomnia or subjective insomnia. It has even been called "pseudo sleep." Patients may complain they did not sleep at all but slept for hours. They may report that they are aware of their surroundings during sleep or are obsessive in thinking during sleep. Bed partners may report they slept soundly or even snored, and others may report they did not seem too sleepy the next day. There is an overestimation of wakefulness during sleep.

It can be distressing and distracting, but usually, those with this disorder actually function reasonably well. It has been linked to metabolism issues, oxygen levels, depression, anxiety, bipolar disorder, alcohol dependency, and stress. During their sleep study, the patient's sleep efficiency will be equal to or over 85%, and they may have slept at least 6.5 hours or more, but in their post-sleep study questionnaire, they report they did not sleep at all or slept very little. There is a mismatch between what we see clinically and what they feel subjectively. It is usually treated with cognitive behavioral therapy, progressive muscle relaxation, stimulus control, exercise, decreased caffeine intake, sleep hygiene, and sometimes medications. We may not understand this disorder completely, and further advancements in our understanding of sleep disorders may shed light on this frustrating disorder.

Alpha Intrusion

Another possibility we see in the sleep lab with PSG examination is "alpha intrusion," a pattern of sleep seen in patients with chronic musculoskeletal pain and other patients with complaints of unrefreshing sleep. It is an abnormal EEG pattern during sleep with alpha waves occurring during delta slow-wave sleep and is associated with non-restorative sleep. Alpha waves usually happen in a relaxed state during the transition from wake to sleep. It has been associated with disorders such as chronic fatigue syndrome, fibromyalgia, anxiety, depression, sleep state misperception, rheumatoid arthritis, thyroid disorders, obstructive sleep apnea, narcolepsy, circadian rhythm disorders, and in patients taking stimulants.

Relationship Stress and Insomnia

Deal with relationship issues earlier in the day and not at bedtime. See a therapist, attend a couple's retreat, start a new activity together, have regularly scheduled date nights, commit to 30 minutes to an hour of alone time together before bedtime to watch a show, talk, go for a walk, have cuddle time, anything with a positive vibe. Do not use that time to argue, discuss bills, or discuss issues with the kids. This is a time to enrich and strengthen your bond. The primary goal is to relax and create a peaceful environment before bedtime.

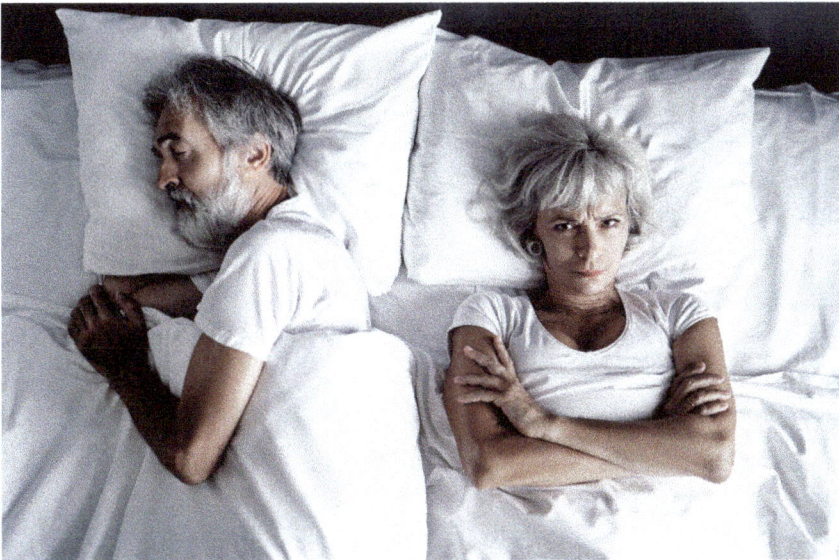

COVID/Long COVID and Sleep

Many infected with COVID have had lingering sleep complaints of insomnia with both initial insomnia and frequent awakenings, fatigue, decreased quantity of sleep, increased napping, and excessive daytime sleepiness being frequent complaints. There are even reports that pre-existing sleep complaints or disorders increased the likelihood of COVID-19, its complications, and the duration of symptoms.

Zhou et al. completed a meta-analysis of forty-eight observational studies demonstrating that pre-existing sleep disturbances increased the risk of COVID-19 susceptibility, hospitalization, mortality, and the development of long COVID-19. These included increased susceptibility and hospitalization in those with obstructive sleep apnea, abnormal sleep duration, and night-shift workers. Mortality from COVID-19 was linked to OSA. The risk of developing long COVID was related to OSA, abnormal sleep duration, and insomnia. Males with a history of sleep disturbances were associated with a higher mortality rate, as was increased age (Zhou et al., 2024).

Batool-Anwar, Fashanu, and Quan reported on 246 patients with severe acute respiratory syndrome coronavirus, and 28% had adverse effects of their sleep lasting beyond twelve months after recovering from the initial infection (Batool-Anwar et al., 2024).

Premraj et al. reviewed 1458 articles, and 19 studies, encompassing a total of 11,324 patients having had COVID, and concluded fatigue, sleep disturbances, and cognitive dysfunction, including brain fog, memory issues, and attention were key features of post-COVID-19 syndrome. Psychiatric manifestations of sleep disturbances, anxiety, and depression increased in prevalence over time (Premraj et al., 2022).

A study out of Vietnam involving 1056 people diagnosed with COVID-19 but not hospitalized for the infection revealed 76% of those patients reported post-COVID insomnia, with 22.8% describing the insomnia as severe. Although insomnia and other significant symptoms occurred in those severe enough to be hospitalized with COVID-19, this study demonstrated insomnia occurred in non-hospitalized COVID-19 patients and asymptomatic COVID-19 patients, too (Hoang et al., 2024).

Donzella revealed sleep patterns among non-hospitalized COVID-19 patients were altered following the infection, regardless of the presentation of symptoms and the time since infection (Donzella et al., 2022).

There have even been reports that COVID-19 may trigger or exacerbate narcolepsy (Roya et al., 2023). As there has long been an autoimmune hypothesis in the development of narcolepsy in some cases, (for example, H1N1 infections and an association with the Pandemrix® vaccination), there is suspicion of similar pathology in post-COVID narcolepsy.

Morelli-Zaher et al. studied 530 patients with post-COVID symptoms. They reported four cases of post-COVID hypersomnia, which were later identified as having idiopathic hypersomnia or type 2 narcolepsy, with three of the patients having a favorable response to methylphenidate. They highlighted the importance of identifying cases of post-COVID central hypersomnia as a treatable symptom (Morelli-Zaher et al., 2024).

So, as you can see above, COVID-19 added a different level of complexity to sleep disorders and symptoms that may need to be considered and treated. We must understand that untreated sleep issues may make one more susceptible to infections and their complications.

Orthosomnia

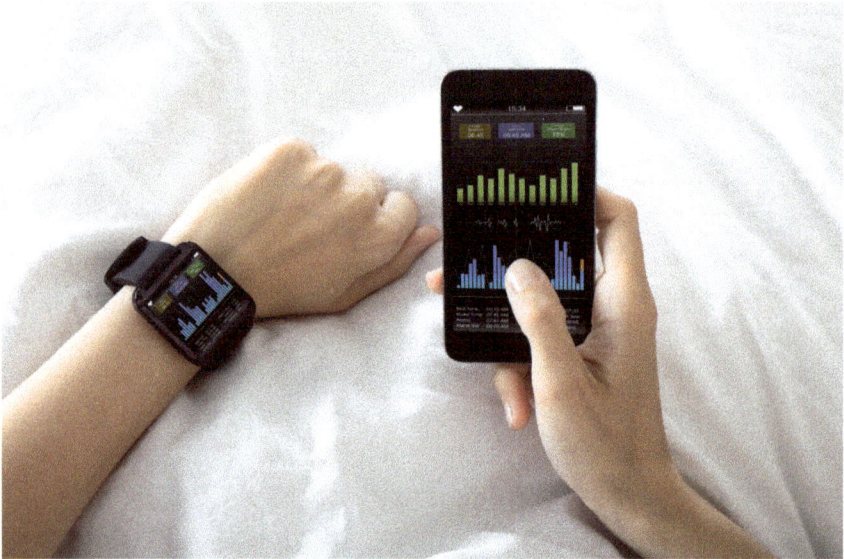

As discussed earlier, orthosomnia is an obsession or preoccupation with obtaining sleep and monitoring it using newer tracking wearable devices or other sleep-tracking technology, such as mobile phones, wearable devices, or even beds now with sleep-tracking reporting.

Patients often predict their next day's performance, mood, and motivation based on how much sleep they think they have gotten. For example, they may wake up and report, "This is going to be a bad day—I did not rest well. My sleep timer told me."

A 2023 article in Nat Sci Sleep entitled "The Tale of Orthosomnia: I Am so Good at Sleeping that I Can Do It with My Eyes Closed and My Fitness Tracker on Me" (Jahrami et al., 2023) describes this struggle. People with this disorder frequently check their sleep trackers and feel anxious if they are separated from their devices. Jahrami and associates discussed the term "Nomophobia" as the fear of not being able to access a mobile phone and its relation to developing orthosomnia so that they can obtain "perfect" sleep. Due to their perception of inadequate sleep and their anxiety about not sleeping well, they may actually develop difficulty falling asleep, frequent awakenings, early morning awakenings, complaints of daytime fatigue or sleepiness, concentration and memory problems, or even anxiety, irritability, and despair. This obsession with monitoring sleep to predict physical and mental well-being can be detrimental.

Two of my patients immediately come to mind who had such a fear of insomnia with such an obsession about their sleep and recording daily outcomes that their whole day was consumed in the preparations of sleep, obsessively talking about their sleep, searching for the perfect mattress or the perfect pillow, depression secondary to the sleep obsession, social isolation, rigid bedtime routines, hyper-focusing on medications in "just the right combo," impaired family or dating relationships, and desperation related to all of the symptoms.

One patient always went to bed by 8 or 8:30 PM to try to get at least eight hours of sleep when they got up at 6:30 AM the following day, with numerous nighttime rituals they repeated to enhance sleep quantity and quality. So, they spent ten hours or more in bed, hoping to get at least eight hours of sleep. This was counterproductive. This behavior resembles a young child trying so hard to ride a bike. You know they can do it, but the harder they try, the more they can't. This may be because they are spending so much of their time in very light or fragmented stage 1 or stage 2 sleep, having issues causing frequent arousals (such as apnea, periodic limb movement disorder, restless legs, significant anxiety, heartburn/reflux, nocturia, or environmental issues) or it could be due to sleep state misperception.

"The day is over; it's time for rest.
Sleep well my dear, you did your best."

~ *Catherine Pulsifer*

Grief and Sleep

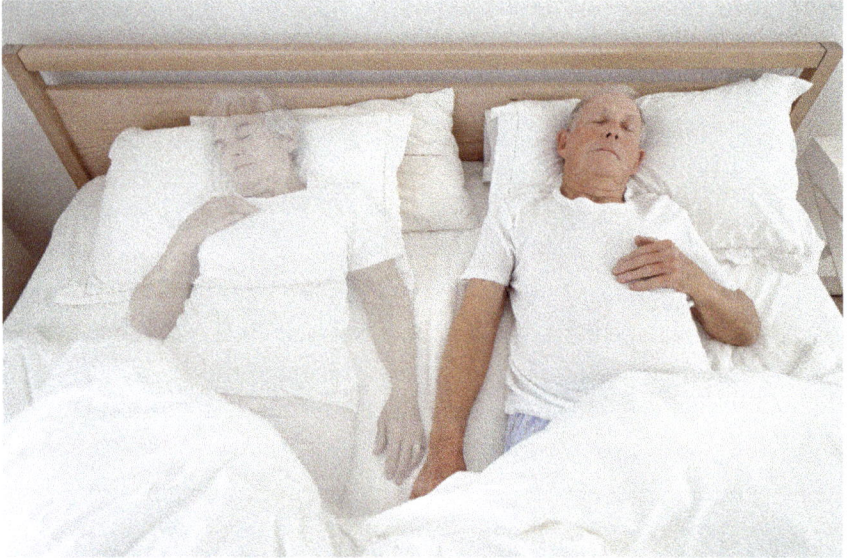

Grief can cause insomnia or even cause patients to stay in bed and sleep too much to avoid thoughts and pain. Grief can occur with the death of a loved one, divorce, or a breakup of a significant relationship. It can occur with the loss of a pet, loss of a job, financial stress, a child leaving home, a miscarriage, retirement, an illness, disability, or injury. Literally, when the heart hurts and one is heartbroken, sleep can be broken. There can be trouble getting to sleep, frequent awakenings, increased dreams or nightmares, and waking unrefreshed. Grief can intensify to a state of full-blown depression, severe anxiety, PTSD, and a multitude of physical or mental disorders. Sleep and grief are bidirectional, meaning they can each make the other worse, creating a vicious cycle. Working on methods to improve sleep may prevent the progression of complicated grief and the disorders mentioned previously. Psychotherapy can be beneficial to both, and cognitive behavioral therapy has long been reported as an effective treatment of insomnia.

Other tips to try include:

- Keep a grief journal that you write in earlier in the day and not at bedtime. For example, "From Grief To Peace" by Heather Stang, M.A. (Stang, 2021).
- Change environmental reminders to create a peaceful and restorative space. Moving the bed around, getting a new comforter set, adding aromatherapy, getting a new mattress, changing the pictures around in the room, or painting the room can signal a new start and not arouse such painful thoughts right before bed.
- Join a grief support group.
- Focus on positive memories in the evening and before bedtime. Think of one specific happy memory and try to remember as many things about the day the picture was taken, such as the light, noise, and smell.
- Do something to honor your loved one.

Treatments for Insomnia

Cognitive behavioral therapy for insomnia is a therapy that is used to address thoughts, behaviors, and actions to improve sleep. It is considered the gold standard of non-pharmacological treatments for insomnia. It involves cognitive therapy, stimulus control, sleep hygiene, relaxation techniques, and mindfulness. It focuses on restructuring faulty thoughts, feelings, and behaviors contributing to insomnia. Examples of some of the steps involved include:

Cognitive Restructuring
- Check your unrealistic sleep expectations and misconceptions about the causes of insomnia.
- Re-evaluate the consequences of sleep deprivation and how you have actually survived and sometimes thrived even if

you have not had a good night's sleep. Predicting you will have a bad day if you do not sleep well will probably make that a reality.

- Performance anxiety can become a sleep issue and contribute to your ongoing insomnia.

Sleep Hygiene
- Regular bedtime
- Regular wake time
- No exercise at least three hours before bedtime
- Avoid nicotine, caffeine, and alcohol three hours before bedtime
- Avoid clock watching

Stimulus Control
- Train to re-associate your bed and bedtime with sleep.
- Limit bed to sleep and sex only. Don't hang out in bed.
- If you are not asleep in 10–20 minutes, get out of bed and do some non-stimulating activity. We want your bed to be a relaxing, pleasant place.

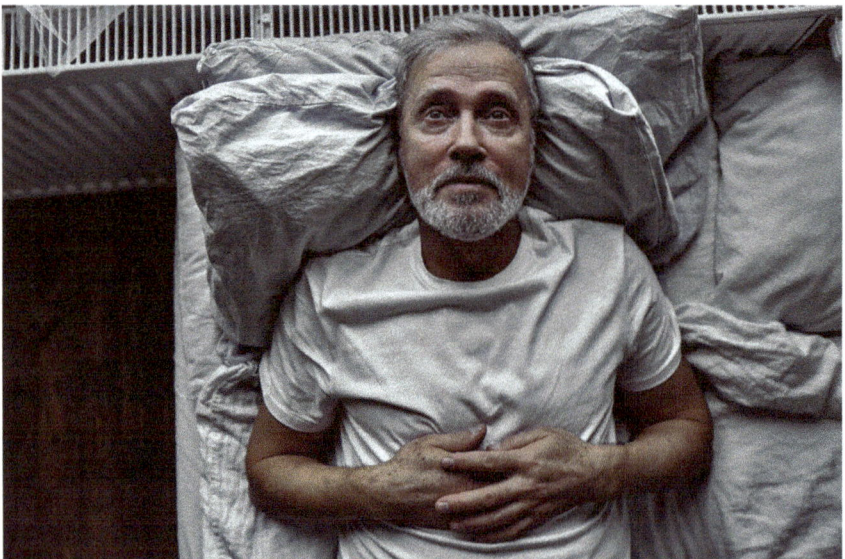

Sleep Restriction
- Use a sleep diary and restrict sleep to a sleep efficiency of 80–90%.
- Not less than four and a half hours.
- Increase by fifteen minutes after the sleep efficiency is >90%.

Relaxation and Biofeedback
- **Progressive muscle relaxation** o This technique involves tensing and then releasing different muscle groups, starting with your toes and moving up your body to your face. You should focus on the tension of the muscle, and then the melting away of relaxation with a long exhale at the end of each muscle group. Relaxing your body and your mind can help promote sleep. There are apps, audio versions, and even videos with instructions to aid you in this process if necessary.
- **Autogenic training** o This desensitization-relaxation technique uses a series of self-statements about heaviness and warmth in different body parts. After getting comfortable and focusing on diaphragmatic breathing from your abdomen with deep breaths to expand your lungs, you focus your mind and body on being calm and relaxed.
- **Imagery training** o This technique uses visualization and mental rehearsal. An example would include a body scan meditation focusing on body parts and their tension and working on releasing tension in each specific area.

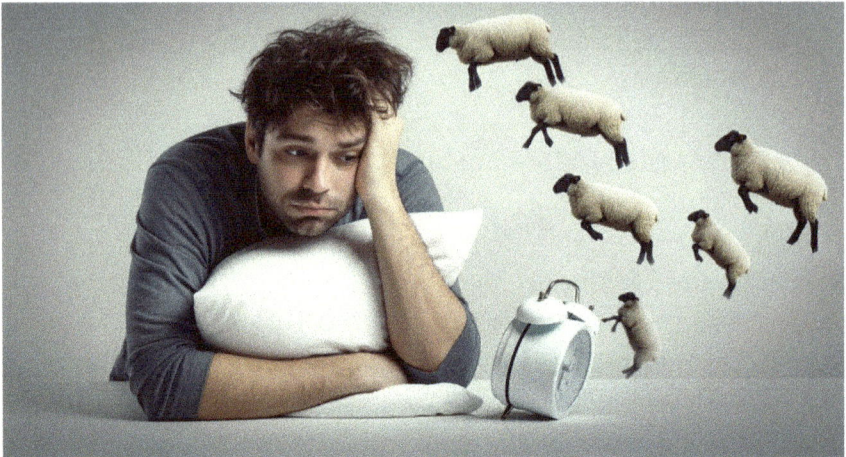

- **Thought stopping** o Thought-stopping involves identifying and redirecting negative thoughts with a more positive thought or behavior. For instance, instead of focusing on "I can't sleep" repeatedly, try distracting yourself from negative thoughts with music, reading a book or magazine, listening to a podcast, doing a puzzle, practicing mindfulness, prayer, doing yoga, or listening to an audiobook. Alternatively, when you catch yourself having a negative thought, you can imagine a stop sign, whisper "stop," write it down, and then write three positive alternative statements to focus on, or try snapping a rubber band on your wrist.
- **Abdominal breathing** o This technique involves placing a hand on your chest and one on your abdomen. While breathing in, focus on expanding your abdomen; while breathing out, allow your abdomen to contract. This can be done at night to help with insomnia or anytime during the day to aid with anxiety and stress.
- **Hypnosis** o Hypnosis creates an altered state of awareness, attention, and a dream-like sensation where one is more open to suggestions used for sleep, smoking, pain, anxiety, insomnia, and various other disorders.

- **Meditation** o Meditation is a deep state of relaxation that allows increased clarity, focus on your attention, and calmness, which promotes a detachment from the mental chaos so often present. With practice, it can help you redirect your thoughts and anxiety.

Paradoxical Intention (PI)
PI is a technique used in cognitive behavioral therapy that encourages patients to intentionally do what they want to avoid. For example, they might be told to stay in bed and stay awake all night. While focusing on performance anxiety as a rate-limiting step in getting to sleep, patients are encouraged to try hard to stay awake and keep their eyes open while lying in a dark room throughout the night.

"Sleep is the best meditation."

~ Dalai Lama

Weighted Blankets

A recent article in the *BMC Psychiatry* (Yu et al., 2024) reported weighted blankets might improve both quality and duration of sleep in people with insomnia. They analyzed 95 adults: 50 with blankets and 45 without. Using the Pittsburgh Sleep Quality Index (PSQI) questionnaire, actigraphy, and other outcomes, they demonstrated improvement on several measures, including their PSQI scores, number of awakenings, daytime sleepiness, fatigue, anxiety, stress, and bodily pain in those who used the blankets.

Some Final Tips

Don't stay in your pajamas or bedclothes during the day, and don't sleep in your sweats or day clothes at night. Putting on pajamas, brushing your teeth, and washing your face should all be a nighttime ritual to signal the start of the sleeping process. Taking pajamas off, brushing your teeth, washing your face, and putting on your daytime clothes help to trigger thoughts of "I am up now; I need to start going for the day."

The above are treatment recommendations specifically for insomnia. Still, the key to treating sleep issues is to examine all potential contributing factors to sleep disruption and address as many problems as possible. The next chapter will provide tips on various topics to consider.

Chapter 13

Sleep Promoting Activities

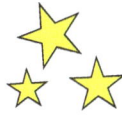

"A well-spent day brings happy sleep."

~ Leonardo da Vinci

So now we have gone over numerous possibilities of things that could be disruptive to your sleep, including your sleep environment, sleeping with pets or your children, your snoring partner, depression, anxiety, pregnancy, hot flashes, Alzheimer's, Parkinson's disease, shift work, substance abuse, alcohol use, caffeine, your weight, nicotine, gastroesophageal reflux, having to go to the bathroom at night, chronic pain, the use of electronics, medications, sleep apnea, narcolepsy, idiopathic hypersomnia, restless legs, nightmares, grinding your teeth, grief, relationship issues, and other things such as a history of COVID. An important thing to realize is that there are often multiple issues at play. Identifying all the factors you may feel are contributing is a priority in ensuring your success in being energized and alert after a restorative night of sleep.

Remember the 3 Ps:

1) Promote healthy sleep with your behavior all day long.
2) Prioritize your sleep.
3) Prepare for bedtime/sleep in the "power hour" before sleep.

A good night's sleep starts first thing in the morning, not just when you lie down at night. Prepare during the day with sunlight exposure, exercise, regulating your emotions, treating underlying psychiatric and medical disorders, organizing your sleep environment, dealing with conflict and stressors earlier in the day, avoiding caffeine after 3 PM, etc.

Make sure you schedule your day to allow enough time to sleep! Don't steal from your sleep and add to your "sleep debt" by waiting too late to pay bills, do laundry, clean the kitchen, do homework, catch up on Netflix, cruise the internet, or return emails. Prioritize your sleep!

Protect the hour before bedtime by turning down the sound on the TV, lowering the lights, taking a hot bath or shower, listening to relaxing music, writing in a gratitude journal, meditating, stretching, focusing on breathing, and spending quality time with your partner or family.

If you can't sleep, get up. The harder you try, the less successful you will be. Next, I will provide tips to help you focus on your sleep that you may need to review periodically to promote healthy restorative sleep.

Stop the Sleep Stealing Tip Sheet

- Think about things you do during the day that may prevent your sleep and make a conscious effort to change them.
- Get daytime sunlight or use a light therapy box earlier in the day. The sunshine and daylight help to set circadian rhythms primarily by regulating melatonin production from the pineal gland in the brain. Morning sunshine decreases melatonin production and, therefore, sleepiness during the day. Daylight exposure has been found to increase sleep duration and improve sleep quality. The CDC reports bright light in the morning will help you fall asleep more easily at night, and avoiding bright light two hours before bedtime will make it easier to fall asleep.
- Check your vitamin D level. Choi al. (2020) reported that "low serum vitamin D status is associated with excessive sleep duration in individuals with low sun exposure. Therefore, in modern society where sun exposure is inevitably low, maintaining an adequate serum vitamin D status may be important for healthy sleep duration."
- Create your "oasis" in your bedroom with a comfortable pillow and mattress, make sure the room is not too hot or too cold, decrease the noise, reduce the light, decrease interruptions, try aroma therapy, reduce the clutter, and create a peaceful place to sleep.
- If your partner snores, ask them to be evaluated for a sleep disorder. Consider a white noise machine or alternate sleeping arrangements if it is severe.
- Use sleep masks if light is an issue in your room.
- Exercise can help improve the deeper restorative stages of slow-wave sleep but should not be done within a few hours of trying to go to sleep.
- Yoga or light stretching in the evening may help relax tension.

- Keep a routine of going to bed and getting up at roughly the same time, even on the weekends.
- Don't nap after 6–7 PM.
- Keep naps short. Set an alarm and sleep for twenty to thirty minutes. Avoid long naps as they can disrupt your sleep later in the evening.
- Schedule a sleep time that gives you seven to eight hours of sleep.
- Plan cuddle time with your partner before your actual desired sleep time.
- Prayer, gratitude journaling, and thinking of happy times may ease your mind and promote sleep.
- Avoid caffeine after 3–5 PM.
- Avoid heavy meals and spicy foods in the evening. Eat dinner earlier and have a light snack before bedtime if needed.
- Treat gastroesophageal reflux with medications or positional therapy to avoid sleep interruptions and sleeping in the lighter stages of sleep.
- Avoid excessive fluids at least three to four hours before bedtime in the evening to prevent frequent bathroom trips.
- Avoid alcohol in the evening. Alcohol can increase sleep apnea, disrupt sleep quality, and increase bathroom trips.
- Avoid nicotine before bedtime, and do not smoke if you wake up in the middle of the night. Nicotine is a stimulant and can delay sleep onset and decrease both the quantity and quality of sleep.
- Start dimming the lights and lowering the TV or music volume one to two hours before sleep.
- Avoid bright lights in the evening and overstimulation.
- Review your evening medications with your physician and/ or pharmacist to see if any of your medications could be contributing to sleep disruption.

- Go to bed only when sleepy.
- Use the bed for sleep, naps, and sex only. Do not work in bed or hang out in bed.
- Take a hot shower or bath one hour before bedtime. Your body temperature, going from very warm to cooling off, helps promote sleep.
- Consider adding Epsom salts to your bath. Epsom salt soaks may help to ease chronic pain, decrease restless legs, reduce stress, and reduce muscle tension. It should be avoided if pregnant or with significantly dry skin.
- Create a "Going to Sleep" song playlist.
- Don't hang out in bed. If you can't get to sleep in about 20 minutes, get up and do some non-stimulating activity, such as flipping through a magazine, watching a light-hearted show, listening to soft music, folding clothes, etc., and then try again later. Do not get on electronics, watch the news, start a movie, or watch an action-packed drama.
- Prayer helps! Turn it over to God or your higher power.
- Mindfulness meditation focuses on the present moment without judgment, paying attention to your breathing, thoughts, and feelings. If your mind gets distracted, gently refocus and bring your attention back to your breathing.
- Focus on your thoughts and feelings and redirect to more positive memories and situations.
- Keep a notebook by your bed to write out any tasks you need to do the next day so that you are not focused on trying to remember them.
- Keep a bottle of water by your bed to sip on if you become thirsty. Don't drink a large volume before bedtime.
- Aromatherapy with lavender.
- Sleep in socks if your feet are cold.
- Wear comfy pajamas. Don't sleep in your sweats or evening clothes. Even the act of changing into bed clothes or taking

off your clothes signals that it is time to switch off and go to sleep.

- Switch off electronics at least 30 minutes before bedtime and silence alerts.
- Commit to only reading 30 minutes or so before bedtime, and don't read an exciting murder mystery or other book you just can't put down.
- Have a light snack, such as milk, bananas, or oatmeal.
- Meditate on sleep quotes (see below).
- Listen to a relaxation program on your phone, CD, or online.
- Visualize your thoughts floating away on balloons from your mind. Let your worries and your troubles float away until tomorrow. Let go of the constant stream of worry and surrender to the present moment.
- Guided imagery or imagery visualization involves imagining yourself in a more relaxed situation and recalling as many details about the situation as possible, including the smells and sounds. For example, imagine a walk in the park—imagine the noise, the feeling of the sunshine on your face, the children playing in the distance, the fragrance of the flowers, the sound of the gravel as you walk, your breathing, etc. There are websites and audio files to help you with these sorts of exercises.
- Progressive muscle relaxation involves permitting yourself to relax, slowing down your breathing, and tensing your muscles for ten to fifteen seconds, then relaxing them for 30 seconds. Start with your toes and work up your body to your head. Then, imagine releasing all the worries, thoughts, and concerns trapped in your brain.
- Remember the 3-2-1 Principle. Stop drinking alcohol for three hours before bed, stop eating two hours before bedtime, and stop drinking fluids one hour before bedtime. Variations include stopping working on stressful activities two hours before bedtime, avoiding electronics one hour

before bedtime, and avoiding smoking four hours before bedtime.

- Don't lie in bed, watching the clock, and count the minutes you have left to sleep if you go to sleep just at that moment. That is torture!
- Don't try so hard!

Quotes for Positivity and Better Sleep

"If you can't sleep, then get up and do something instead of lying there worrying. It's the worry that gets you, not the lack of sleep."

~ Dale Carnegie

"Man should forget his anger before lying down to sleep."

~ Mahatma Gandhi

"Watch your thoughts, they become your words; watch your words, they become your actions; watch your actions, they become your habits; watch your habits, they become your character; watch your character, it becomes your destiny."

~ Lao Tzu

"Change your thoughts, and you change your world."

~ Norman Vincent Peale

"Thinking will not overcome fear, but action will."

~ W. Clement Stone

"You have two choices: to control your mind or to let your mind control you."

~ Paulo Coelho

"Once you replace negative thoughts with positive ones, you'll start having positive results."

~ Willie Nelson

"Nothing in life is quite as important as you think it is while you're thinking about it."

~ Daniel Kahneman

"The greatest discovery of my generation is that a human being can alter his life by altering his attitudes of mind."

~ William James

"It's only a thought, and a thought can be changed."

~ Louise Hay

"Many things—such as loving, going to sleep, or behaving unaffectedly—are done worst when we try hardest to do them."

~ C.S. Lewis

"Be aware of your breathing. Notice how this takes attention away from your thinking and creates space."

~ Eckhart Tolle

"Let Gratitude be the pillow upon which you kneel to say your nightly prayer."

~ Maya Angelou

"Put your thoughts to sleep; do not cast a shadow over the moon of your heart. Let go of thinking."

~ Rumi (Persian poet)

"Sleep is an investment in the energy you need to be effective tomorrow."

~ Tom Roth

"Your future depends on your dreams, so go to sleep."

~ Mesut Barazany

"Get some sleep.

It's in my hands."

~ God

Facebook post

"When you lie down, you will not be afraid; when you lie down, your sleep will be sweet."

~ Proverbs 3:24

Chapter 14

Conclusion —
Your Sleep Matters!

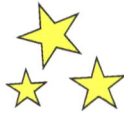

"No one cares how much you know until they know how much you care."

~ Theodore Roosevelt

I hope you now understand how much I sincerely care about sharing information on the importance of sleep and how much I hope you will also care about and prioritize your sleep, incorporating some of these ideas into your lifestyle. As I have said before, sleep is a foundation of your physical and mental well-being. A good night's sleep can help overwhelming things seem manageable. It can improve immunity, mental health, physical health, relationships, academic or occupational performance, and concentration/memory, and it can help prevent other disorders from developing.

Remember the 3 Ps of Sleep:

1) Prioritize sleep.
2) Promote healthy sleep habits.
3) Prepare during the power hour before sleep!

List your goals for the next month, three months, six months, and the following year you hope to achieve by addressing your sleep issues, and write them down to help you manifest these outcomes. Post them somewhere in your house so you'll see them often. Pick three things to try at a time. Document what is successful in a journal or notebook so that if you need to refer to it in the future, you will be reminded of what made a difference. Additionally, various factors may work for you at different times, depending on your stressors, medical issues, environmental conditions, and other relevant considerations. Refer back to the tips provided in this book when necessary. Retake the sleep questionnaire occasionally to see if your priorities have changed. Please make a list of concerns and share them with your provider. Alert others to your sleep-prioritizing plans so they can support your success and respect the goals and boundaries you are setting. Reset and readjust as needed.

You are a priority, your sleep is a priority, and your health is a priority!

Sweet dreams,

Debra J. Stultz, MD

"Day is over, night has come. Today is gone, what's done is done. Embrace your dreams through the night. Tomorrow comes with a whole new light."

~ George Orwell

References

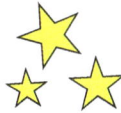

American Psychiatric Association. (2013). *Diagnostic and statistical manual of mental disorders*. American Psychiatric Association. https://doi.org/10.1176/appi.books.9780890425596

Baron, K. G., Abbott, S., Jao, N., Manalo, N., & Mullen, R. (2017). Orthosomnia: Are some patients taking the quantified self too far? *Journal of Clinical Sleep Medicine*, *13*(02), 351–354. https://doi.org/10.5664/jcsm.6472

Batool-Anwar, S., Fashanu, O. S., & Quan, S. F. (2024). Long-term effects of COVID-19 on sleep patterns. *Thoracic Research and Practice*. https://doi.org/10.5152/ThoracResPract.2024.24013

Choi, J. H., Lee, B., Lee, J. Y., Kim, C.-H., Park, B., Kim, D. Y., Kim, H. J., & Park, D.-Y. (2020). Relationship between sleep duration, sun exposure, and serum 25-hydroxyvitamin D status: A cross-sectional study. *Scientific Reports*, *10*(1), 4168. https://doi.org/10.1038/s41598-020-61061-8

Daldoul, A., Ammar, N., Krir, M. W., Khechine, W., Hajji, A., Bergaoui, H., Ghazouani, N., Migaou, H., Zaied, S., & Zoukar, O. (2023). Insomnia in breast cancer: Prevalence and associated factors. In *BMJ Supportive and Palliative Care* (Vol. 13, Issue e1, pp. E51–E52). BMJ Publishing Group. https://doi.org/10.1136/bmjspcare-2020-002718

Dauvilliers, Y., Bogan, R. K., Arnulf, I., Scammell, T. E., St Louis, E. K., & Thorpy, M. J. (2022). Clinical considerations for the diagnosis of idiopathic hypersomnia. *Sleep Medicine Reviews, 66,* 101709. https://doi.org/10.1016/j.smrv.2022.101709

Davis, J. L., & Wright, D. C. (2006). Exposure, relaxation, and rescripting treatment for trauma-related nightmares. *Journal of Trauma & Dissociation, 7*(1), 5–18. https://doi.org/10.1300/J229v07n01_02

Dilanardo, M. J. (2024, April 11). The connection between sleep and obesity. WebMD. https://www.webmd.com/sleepdisorders/sleep-obesisty

Donzella, S. M., Kohler, L. N., Crane, T. E., Jacobs, E. T., Ernst, K. C., Bell, M. L., Catalfamo, C. J., Begay, R., Pogreba-Brown, K., & Farland, L. V. (2022). COVID-19 infection, the COVID-19 pandemic, and changes in sleep. *Frontiers in Public Health, 9.* https://doi.org/10.3389/fpubh.2021.795320

Drake, C., Roehrs, T., Shambroom, J., & Roth, T. (2013). Caffeine effects on sleep taken 0, 3, or 6 hours before going to bed. *Journal of Clinical Sleep Medicine, 09*(11), 1195–1200. https://doi.org/10.5664/jcsm.3170

Finan, P. H., Goodin, B. R., & Smith, M. T. (2013). The association of sleep and pain: An update and a path forward. *The Journal of Pain, 14*(12), 1539–1552. https://doi.org/10.1016/j.jpain.2013.08.007

Gardiner, C., Weakley, J., Burke, L. M., Roach, G. D., Sargent, C., Maniar, N., Townshend, A., & Halson, S. L. (2023). The effect of caffeine on subsequent sleep: A systematic review and meta-analysis. *Sleep Medicine Reviews, 69,* 101764. https://doi.org/10.1016/j.smrv.2023.101764

Grau-López, L., Grau-López, L., Daigre, C., Palma-Álvarez, R. F., Martínez-Luna, N., Ros-Cucurull, E., Ramos-Quiroga, J. A., & Roncero, C. (2020). Insomnia symptoms in patients with substance use disorders during detoxification and associated clinical features. *Frontiers in Psychiatry, 11.* https://doi.org/10.3389/fpsyt.2020.540022

He, S., Hasler, B. P., & Chakravorty, S. (2019). Alcohol and sleep-related problems. *Current Opinion in Psychology, 30,* 117–122. https://doi.org/10.1016/j.copsyc.2019.03.007

Hoang, H. T. X., Yeung, W. F., Truong, Q. T. M., Le, C. T., Bui, A. T. M., Bui, Q. V., Le, Q. T. Le, & Quach, L. H. (2024). Sleep quality among non-hospitalized COVID-19 survivors: A national cross-sectional study. *Frontiers in Public Health, 11*. https://doi.org/10.3389/fpubh.2023.1281012

Holzinger, B., Saletu, B., & Klösch, G. (2020). Cognitions in sleep: Lucid dreaming as an intervention for nightmares in patients with posttraumatic stress disorder. *Frontiers in Psychology, 11*. https://doi.org/10.3389/fpsyg.2020.01826

Howell, M., Avidan, A. Y., Foldvary-Schaefer, N., Malkani, R. G., During, E. H., Roland, J. P., McCarter, S. J., Zak, R. S., Carandang, G., Kazmi, U., & Ramar, K. (2023). Management of REM sleep behavior disorder: An American Academy of Sleep Medicine clinical practice guideline. *Journal of Clinical Sleep Medicine, 19*(4), 759–768. https://doi.org/10.5664/jcsm.10424

Jahrami, H., Trabelsi, K., Husain, W., Ammar, A., BaHammam, A. S., Pandi-Perumal, S. R., Saif, Z., & Vitiello, M. V. (2024). Prevalence of orthosomnia in a general population sample: A cross-sectional study. *Brain Sciences, 14*(11), 1123. https://doi.org/10.3390/brainsci14111123

Jahrami, H., Trabelsi, K., Vitiello, M. V, & BaHammam, A. S. (2023). The tale of orthosomnia: I am so good at sleeping that I can do it with my eyes closed and my fitness tracker on me. *Nature and Science of Sleep, Volume 15*, 13–15. https://doi.org/10.2147/NSS.S402694

Khan I, S. J. (2025). Exploding head syndrome. *StatPearls*. https://www.ncbi.nlm.nih.gov/books/NBK560817/publishing

Kuang, B., Li, D., Lobbezoo, F., de Vries, R., Hilgevoord, A., de Vries, N., Huynh, N., Lavigne, G., & Aarab, G. (2022). Associations between sleep bruxism and other sleep-related disorders in adults: A systematic review. *Sleep Medicine, 89*, 31–47. https://doi.org/10.1016/j.sleep.2021.11.008

Lancee, J., Effting, M., & Kunze, A. E. (2021). Telephone-guided imagery rehearsal therapy for nightmares: Efficacy and mediator of change. *Journal of Sleep Research, 30*(3). https://doi.org/10.1111/jsr.13123

Lunsford-Avery, J. R., Carskadon, M. A., Kollins, S. H., & Krystal, A. D. (2025). Sleep hysiology and neurocognition among adolescents with attention-deficit/hyperactivity disorder. *Journal of the American Academy of Child & Adolescent Psychiatry, 64*(2), 276–289. https://doi.org/10.1016/j.jaac.2024.03.005

McBeth, J., Dixon, W. G., Moore, S. M., Hellman, B., James, B., Kyle, S. D., Lunt, M., Cordingley, L., Yimer, B. B., & Druce, K. L. (2022). Sleep disturbance and quality of life in rheumatoid arthritis: Prospective health study. *Journal of Medical Internet Research, 24*(4), e32825. https://doi.org/10.2196/32825

Morelli-Zaher, C., Vremaroiu-Coman, A., Coquoz, N., Genecand, L., Altarelli, M., Binkova, A., Frésard, I., Bridevaux, P.-O., & Gex, G. (2024). Post-COVID central hypersomnia, a treatable trait in long COVID: 4 case reports. *Frontiers in Neurology, 15*. https://doi.org/10.3389/fneur.2024.1349486

Morgenthaler, T. I., Auerbach, S., Casey, K. R., Kristo, D., Maganti, R., Ramar, K., Zak, R., & Kartje, R. (2018). Position paper for the treatment of nightmare disorder in adults: An American Academy of Sleep Medicine position paper. *Journal of Clinical Sleep Medicine, 14*(06), 1041–1055. https://doi.org/10.5664/jcsm.7178

Mork, P. J., & Nilsen, T. I. L. (2012). Sleep problems and risk of fibromyalgia: Longitudinal data on an adult female population in Norway. *Arthritis & Rheumatism, 64*(1), 281–284. https://doi.org/10.1002/art.33346

Nuñez, A., Rhee, J. U., Haynes, P., Chakravorty, S., Patterson, F., Killgore, W. D. S., Gallagher, R. A., Hale, L., Branas, C., Carrazco, N., Alfonso-Miller, P., Gehrels, J.-A., & Grandner, M. A. (2021). Smoke at night and sleep worse? The associations between cigarette smoking with insomnia severity and sleep duration. *Sleep Health, 7*(2), 177–182. https://doi.org/10.1016/j.sleh.2020.10.006

O'Callaghan, F., Muurlink, O., & Reid, N. (2018). Effects of caffeine on sleep quality and daytime functioning. *Risk Management and Healthcare Policy, Volume 11*, 263–271. https://doi.org/10.2147/RMHP.S156404

Orbeta, R. L., Overpeck, M. D., Ramcharran, D., Kogan, M. D., & Ledsky, R. (2006). High caffeine intake in adolescents: Associations with difficulty sleeping and feeling tired in the morning. *Journal of Adolescent Health, 38*(4), 451–453. https://doi.org/10.1016/j.jadohealth.2005.05.014

Peracchia, S., & Curcio, G. (2018). Exposure to video games: Effects on sleep and on post-sleep cognitive abilities. A systematic review of experimental evidences. *Sleep Science, 11*(04), 302–314. https://doi.org/10.5935/1984-0063.20180046

Premraj, L., Kannapadi, N. V., Briggs, J., Seal, S. M., Battaglini, D., Fanning, J., Suen, J., Robba, C., Fraser, J., & Cho, S.-M. (2022). Mid and long-term neurological and neuropsychiatric manifestations of post-COVID-19 syndrome: A meta-analysis. *Journal of the Neurological Sciences, 434,* 120162. https://doi.org/10.1016/j.jns.2022.120162

Robbins, R., Quan, S. F., Weaver, M. D., Bormes, G., Barger, L. K., & Czeisler, C. A. (2021). Examining sleep deficiency and disturbance and their risk for incident dementia and all-cause mortality in older adults across 5 years in the United States. *Aging, 13*(3), 3254–3268. https://doi.org/10.18632/aging.202591

Roya, Y., Farzaneh, B., Mostafa, A., Mahsa, S., & Babak, Z. (2023). Narcolepsy following COVID-19: A case report and review of potential mechanisms. *Clinical Case Reports, 11*(6). https://doi.org/10.1002/ccr3.7370

Sepkowitz, K. A. (2013). Energy drinks and caffeine-related adverse effects. *JAMA, 309*(3), 243. https://doi.org/10.1001/jama.2012.173526

Van Looveren, E., Bilterys, T., Munneke, W., Cagnie, B., Ickmans, K., Mairesse, O., Malfliet, A., De Baets, L., Nijs, J., Goubert, D., Danneels, L., Moens, M., & Meeus, M. (2021). The association between sleep and chronic spinal pain: A systematic review from the last decade. *Journal of Clinical Medicine, 10*(17), 3836. https://doi.org/10.3390/jcm10173836

Wennberg, A., Wu, M., Rosenberg, P., & Spira, A. (2017). Sleep disturbance, cognitive decline, and dementia: A review. *Seminars in Neurology, 37*(04), 395–406. https://doi.org/10.1055/s-00371604351

Whale, K., & Gooberman-Hill, R. (2022). The importance of sleep for people with chronic pain: Current insights and evidence. *JBMR Plus, 6*(7). https://doi.org/10.1002/jbm4.10658

Yu, J., Du, J., Yang, Z., Chen, W., Sun, S., Gan, M., Cai, Y., Zhang, L., Sun, K., Xu, J., Xu, Q., Ke, J., Zhang, L., Zhu, Y., & Liu, Z. (2024). Effect of weighted blankets on sleep quality among adults with insomnia: A pilot randomized controlled trial. *BMC Psychiatry, 24*(1), 765. https://doi.org/10.1186/s12888-024-06218-9

Zhou, J., Li, X., Zhang, T., Liu, Z., Li, P., Yu, N., & Wang, W. (2024). Pre-existing sleep disturbances and risk of COVID-19: A meta-analysis. *EClinicalMedicine, 74,* 102719. https://doi.org/10.1016/j.eclinm.2024.102719

Zwyghuizen-Doorenbos, A., Roehrs, T. A., Lipschutz, L., Timms, V., & Roth, T. (1990). Effects of caffeine on alertness. *Psychopharmacology*, *100*(1), 36–39. https://doi.org/10.1007/BF02245786

Appendix 1

Stultz Sleep and Behavioral Health

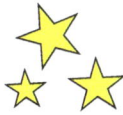

★★★

Intake Evaluation

Presenting problem: *(include present symptoms, their duration, precipitating events, and any past history of these symptoms)*

_____

_____

_____

_____

_____

_____

Have you ever seen a therapist or psychiatrist for these complaints? If so, please list the provider's name, the treatment offered, and your response to that treatment.

_____

_____

_____

_____

_____

Please list your current physicians:

_____

_____

_____

_____

Please select an answer:

Are you satisfied with your sleep?	☐ YES	☐ NO
Have you been feeling depressed?	☐ YES	☐ NO

If yes, how long have you felt depressed?

    ☐ < 3 months
    ☐ 3-6 months
    ☐ > 1 year
    ☐ > 2 years

Have you had more than one episode of depression?	☐ YES	☐ NO
Have you been having mood swings that occur out of the blue?	☐ YES	☐ NO
Have you been feeling nervous or anxious?	☐ YES	☐ NO
Have you been having anxiety attacks?	☐ YES	☐ NO
Are you satisfied with your sex life?	☐ YES	☐ NO
Have you been concerned about your weight?	☐ YES	☐ NO

Have you ever had a head injury with loss of consciousness?	☐ YES	☐ NO
Do you have problems with insomnia?	☐ YES	☐ NO
Has anyone ever told you that you snore?	☐ YES	☐ NO
Do you have trouble with excessive daytime sleepiness?	☐ YES	☐ NO
Do you have trouble with restless legs at night?	☐ YES	☐ NO
Does your bed partner (or parent, if child) complain about your sleep?	☐ YES	☐ NO
Do you have problems with chronic pain?	☐ YES	☐ NO
Are you on any over-the-counter medications regularly?	☐ YES	☐ NO
Is there any chance you may be pregnant?	☐ YES	☐ NO
Have you had laboratory tests done in the past 6 months?	☐ YES	☐ NO
If so, where? _____		
Have you ever had a seizure?	☐ YES	☐ NO
Do you have problems with anxiety in social situations?	☐ YES	☐ NO
Have you ever been diagnosed with ADHD?	☐ YES	☐ NO
Do you suffer from migraines?	☐ YES	☐ NO
Do you have a history of chronic pain?	☐ YES	☐ NO
Have you ever attempted suicide?	☐ YES	☐ NO

Please mark any symptoms you have been experiencing:

☐ Decreased sleep

☐ Increased sleep

☐ Decreased appetite

☐ Increased appetite

☐ Decreased energy

☐ Increased energy

☐ Decrease in concentration

☐ Decreased memory

☐ Increased tearfulness

☐ Decreased interests

☐ Decreased motivation

☐ Trouble making decisions

☐ Indecisiveness

☐ Reduced sex drive

☐ Increased sex drive

☐ Decreased self-esteem

☐ Hopelessness

☐ Helplessness

☐ Thoughts of suicide

☐ Dry mouth

☐ Trembling

☐ Numbness and tingling

☐ Feeling as if you have a lump in your throat

☐ Increased heart rate

☐ Feeling as if your heart skips beats

☐ Chest pains

☐ Shortness of breath

☐ Nausea/Vomiting

☐ Diarrhea

☐ Increased urination

☐ Muscle twitching/cramps

☐ Muscle tension

☐ Hot flashes or chills

☐ Worrying constantly

☐ Fear of crowds, public places, or driving

☐ Being a perfectionist

☐ Checking or re-checking things

☐ Rituals you must complete

☐ Thoughts of hurting others

☐ Hallucinations

☐ Suspiciousness/paranoia

☐ Worthlessness

☐ Increased feelings of guilt

☐ Mood swings

☐ Irritable mood

☐ Impulsive behavior

☐ Increased talkativeness

☐ Hypersexual activity

☐ Increased aggression

☐ Spending sprees

☐ Racing thoughts

☐ Dizziness or lightheadedness

☐ Superstitious thoughts

☐ Frequent handwashing

☐ Fear of germs

☐ Unwanted thoughts

☐ OCD symptoms

☐ Concerns about your weight

☐ Concerns about your appearance

☐ Skipping meals to lose weight

☐ Excessive eating

☐ Making yourself throw up after eating

☐ Using diet pills

☐ Using laxatives

☐ Using water pills or diuretics

☐ Exercising excessively

If you have a history of **migraines**, please check the following treatments you have tried:

☐ Over-the-counter meds

☐ Imitrex (sumatriptan)

☐ Maxalt (rizatriptan)

☐ Axert (almotriptan)

☐ Amerge (naratriptan)

☐ Froza (frozatriptan)

☐ Topomax (topiramate)

☐ Treximet (sumatriptan naproxen)

☐ Cafergot (ergotamine/ caffeine)

☐ Reglan (metoclopramide)

☐ Inderal (propranolol)

☐ Zestril (lisinopril)

☐ Migergot (ergotamine/ caffeine)

☐ Nurtec (rimegepant)

☐ Ubrelvy (ubrogepant)

☐ Botox (onabotulinumtoxinA)

☐ Opioids/pain meds/ narcotics

☐ ER trips due to migraine

☐ Missed work/school due to the migraine

☐ Zomig (zolmitriptan)

☐ Relpax (eletriptan)

☐ Depakote (divalproex sodium)

☐ Steroids (prednisone dexamethasone)

☐ Migranal (DHE)

☐ Zofran (ondansetron)

☐ Isoptin or Calan (verapamil)

☐ Antidepressants

☐ Elavil (amitriptyline)

☐ Effexor (venlafaxine)

☐ Cymbalta (duloxetine)

Please list any other symptoms you are concerned about:

_____

_____

_____

_____

Past medical history: *(please list any current medical problems, as well as past medical problems)*

_____

_____

_____

_____

Past history of surgery: *(please list any surgeries)*

_____

_____

_____

_____

Current medications: *(list names, dosages, and how often you take them; include over-the-counter medicines that you take)*

_____

_____

_____

_____

_____

_____

_____

_____

_____

_____

_____

_____

_____

Drug allergies: *(Please name the drug and the reaction)*

_____

_____

_____

Family medical history: *(please list any illness of any blood relatives, including such illnesses as heart disease, strokes, diabetes, thyroid problems, cancer, high blood pressure, lung disease, kidney disease, seizures, sleep apnea, narcolepsy, restless legs syndrome, etc.)*

_____

_____

_____

Family psychiatric history: *(please include any illness of any blood relatives, including such problems as depression, nervousness, mood swings, heavy alcohol or drug use, nervous breakdown, or suicide)*

_____

_____

_____

_____

Social History:

How many siblings do you have? _____

Any history of physical/sexual/emotional abuse? _____

Years of education: _____

Sexual orientation: _____

Gender identity: _____

Marital status: _____

How many times have you been married? _____

Any history of domestic violence? _____

Legal history? _____

DUI arrest? _____

How many children do you have? _____

What is your religious/spiritual preference? _____

What is your occupation? _____

Are there any other stressors that you have been concerned about?

_____

_____

_____

_____

_____

_____

_____

_____

Name three (3) things that you enjoy doing:

_____

_____

_____

Please Answer:

Your height: _____

Your weight: _____

Have you ever received substance abuse treatment? ☐ YES ☐ NO

How many days a month do you drink alcohol? _____

How much do you drink over one of these days? _____

Are you currently on or have you been prescribed Methadone or Suboxone? ☐ YES ☐ NO

Are you currently prescribed opioids/narcotics? ☐ YES ☐ NO

How much nicotine do you smoke or vape? _____

How many other drugs do you smoke or vape? _____

When it comes to alcohol or illegal/illicit drugs, which have you used regularly, now or in the past?

_____

_____

_____

_____

What problems have these caused in your life?

_____

_____

_____

_____

How do you exercise, and how often? _____

_____

Do you feel you have a problem with your weight? ☐ YES ☐ NO

If so, please complete the following questions:

____ I have been binge eating at least once a week for the last three months

____ I feel powerless to prevent a binge

____ I feel powerless to stop a binge once it has started

____ My binges last no more than two hours and occasionally in more than one sitting

____ I usually binge alone because I don't want others to see me

____ I eat very fast during a binge

____ I keep eating even if I am full

____ I binge even though I am not hungry

____ I will binge on just about any food

____ I have gone out to buy food, even at odd hours, when I feel a binge coming on

____ After a binge, I feel terrible—depressed, disgusted, ashamed, guilty, out of control

____ During a binge, I feel like I am "zoning out."

____ I do not try to "undo" my binges by vomiting, taking laxatives, or exercising excessively

____ I am distressed about my binging and feel as if I am caught in a vicious cycle

<u>Sleep Questionnaire</u>

Please describe your current sleep complaints and what may make them better or worse:

_____

_____

_____

_____

_____

Have you had a prior sleep study? If so, when and where:

_____

_____

<u>Please answer:</u>

Have you ever been diagnosed with obstructive sleep apnea?	☐YES	☐NO
Do you wear oxygen or use a CPAP or BIPAP?	☐YES	☐NO
Has anyone ever complained about your sleeping habits or your behavior during sleep? *(insomnia, restlessness, snoring, sleep schedule, kicking, sleep talking, etc.)*	☐YES	☐NO

Do you have problems with insomnia or trouble getting to sleep?	☐YES	☐NO
Do you have problems staying asleep?	☐YES	☐NO
Do you have problems with awakening earlier than you had planned?	☐YES	☐NO

What interventions have you tried to help with your insomnia? Describe medications and behaviors.

_____

_____

_____

How many hours of sleep do you get? During the week: _____
Weekends: _____

How many hours of sleep do you need to feel rested? _____

Do you snore?	☐YES	☐NO
Have you ever been told that you stop breathing or have pauses in your breathing while you are sleeping?	☐YES	☐NO
Are you an active sleeper? (Waken with your bedclothes in disarray?)	☐YES	☐NO
Do you sweat excessively at night?	☐YES	☐NO
Do you wake up gasping, choking, or feeling short of breath?	☐YES	☐NO

Do you work split or rotation shifts?

How often do you take naps?

More than once a day:	☐
At least once a day:	☐
A few times per week:	☐
Rarely:	☐

How do you feel after taking a nap?

Very refreshed:	☐
Somewhat refreshed:	☐
Somewhat tired:	☐
Very drowsy:	☐

Have you ever had a sudden, irresistible attack of sleep? ☐YES ☐NO

Do you lose muscle strength when you experience intense emotions such as laughing, anger, surprise, sadness, or happiness? (example: weakness in your knees, sagging facial muscles, blurred vision, slurred speech, clumsiness, dropping things, falls, neck/shoulder weakness or complete collapse) ☐YES ☐NO

Do you experience episodes when you are going to sleep or awakening in which you briefly feel paralyzed? ☐YES ☐NO

Do you ever experience hearing or seeing something that is not real as you are going to or coming from sleep? ☐YES ☐NO

Do you have vivid dreams or nightmares? ☐YES ☐NO

Is there anything in your environment that may contribute to your sleep disruption? (example: your bed partner, pets in the room, temperature extremes, small children, noise, lights, or an uncomfortable mattress) ☐YES ☐NO

If so, explain:

_____

_____

_____

Do you have to get up at night to go to the bathroom? ☐ YES   ☐ NO

If so, how many times a night? _____

Do you have an unpleasant sensation in your legs, such as restless legs, a crawling sensation, an aching sensation, or an inability to keep your legs still? ☐ YES   ☐ NO

Have you ever been told that you kick in your sleep? ☐ YES   ☐ NO

Do you experience any pain or discomfort that may ☐ YES   ☐ NO be contributing to your sleep disturbance? If so, explain:

_____

_____

Do you have any family members with a history of sleep disorders?
☐ YES   ☐ NO

(Sleep apnea, narcolepsy, or "sleepy heads," ☐ YES   ☐ NO restless legs, insomnia, snoring) If so, explain:

_____

_____

Is there any other information you feel may help evaluate your sleep complaints?

_____

_____

_____

Do you have problems with any of the following symptoms? Place an 'X' beside all that apply:

☐ Racing thoughts at night

☐ Chronic pain

☐ Talking during your sleep

☐ Waking with an acid or sour taste in your mouth

☐ Waking/screaming/fearful in the first third of the night

☐ History of seizures

☐ Unusual or violent movements during your sleep

☐ Periods of inappropriate eating before sleep

☐ Muscle tension

☐ Fearful about your inability to sleep

☐ Grinding your teeth at night

☐ Unusual movement in your sleep

☐ History of bedwetting as a child

☐ Sleepwalking

☐ Problems with impotence or sexual dysfunction

For Males:

☐ History of low testosterone

☐ Sexual dysfunction

☐ Painful erections that awaken you

Do you have a history of:

☐ Stroke

☐ Seizure

☐ Asthma

☐ COPD

☐ Heart disease

☐ Decreased memory

☐ Hypertension

☐ Oxygen use

Restless Legs:

Please check any of the following symptoms you have:

- ☐ A strong urge to move legs, feet, or arms due to an uncomfortable sensation.
- ☐ Discomfort that is relieved by movement that reoccurs when the movement ends
- ☐ Symptoms are activated by rest or relaxation and during sleep
- ☐ Symptoms become worse at night and subside in the morning. Do these occur in your:
  - ☐ Arms ☐ Day ☐ Sleep
  - ☐ Legs ☐ Night

Bed Partner Questionnaire

Patient's name: _____ Date: _____

Your name: _____

Please Circle the Correct Answer:

Does your bed partner snore? ☐ Never ☐ Occasionally ☐ Often

In which position does your bed partner snore?
☐ Back ☐ Side ☐ Stomach ☐ All positions

Is this worse with alcohol intake? ☐ YES   ☐ NO

How much and how often does your bed partner consume alcohol?

_____

Have you noticed your bed partner has pauses in their breathing or other abnormal breathing patterns during sleep? ☐ YES ☐ NO

Please select any of the following behaviors you have observed in your bed partner's sleep:

☐ Sleepwalking   ☐ Gasping

☐ Sleep talking   ☐ Kicking

☐ Violent movements   ☐ Grinding teeth

☐ Gagging   ☐ Moving legs excessively before sleep

☐ Choking   ☐ Napping during the day

☐ Snorting   ☐ Falling asleep unintentionally

Are there any other unusual behaviors associated with your bed partner's sleep or other information you feel may be helpful?

_____

_____

_____

_____

_____

_____

Please mark any of the medications you have previously tried or are currently taking:

- ☐ Anafranil (Clomipramine)
- ☐ Celexa (Citalopram)
- ☐ Cymbalta (Duloxetine)
- ☐ Effexor (Venlafaxine)
- ☐ Elavil (Amitriptyline)
- ☐ Fetzima (Levomilnacipran)
- ☐ Lexapro (Escitalopram)
- ☐ Luvox (Fluvoxamine)
- ☐ Luvox CR
- ☐ Norpramin (Desipramine)
- ☐ Nuedexta (Dextromethorphan/ Quinidine)
- ☐ Pamelor (Nortriptyline)
- ☐ Paxil (Paroxetine)
- ☐ Paxil CR
- ☐ Pexeva (Paroxetine)
- ☐ Pristiq (Desvenlafaxine)
- ☐ Prozac (Fluoxetine)
- ☐ Remeron (Mirtazapine)
- ☐ Serzone (Nefazodone)
- ☐ Sinequan (Doxepin)
- ☐ Tofranil (Imipramine)
- ☐ Trintellix (Vortioxetine)
- ☐ Viibryd (Vilazodone)
- ☐ Wellbutrin (Bupropion)
- ☐ Zoloft (Sertraline)

****

- ☐ Abilify (Aripiprazole)

- ☐ Chlorpromazine (Thorazine)
- ☐ Depakote/Depakene (Valproic Acid)
- ☐ Fanapt (Iloperidone)
- ☐ Geodon (Ziprasidone)
- ☐ Haldol (Haloperidol)
- ☐ Invega (Paliperidone)
- ☐ Keppra (Levetiracetam)
- ☐ Lamictal (Lamotrigine)
- ☐ Latuda (Lurasidone)
- ☐ Lithium (Lithane, Lithobid)
- ☐ Loxitane (Loxapine)
- ☐ Navane (Thiothixene)
- ☐ Neurontin (Gabapentin)
- ☐ Rexulti (Brexpiprazole)
- ☐ Risperdal (Risperidone)
- ☐ Saphris (Asenapine)
- ☐ Seroquel (Quetiapine)
- ☐ Seroquel XR
- ☐ Stavzor (Valproic acid)
- ☐ Symbyax (Fluoxetine/ Olanzapine)
- ☐ Topomax (Topiramate)
- ☐ Trileptal (Oxcarbazepine)
- ☐ Vraylar (Cariprazine)
- ☐ Stavzor (Valproic Acid)
- ☐ Zyprexa (Olanzapine)

****

- ☐ Ambien (Zolpidem)
- ☐ Ambien CR

- ☐ Belsomra (Suvorexant)
- ☐ Clonidine
- ☐ Halcion (Triazolam)
- ☐ Intermezzo (Zolpidem)
- ☐ Lunesta (Eszopiclone)
- ☐ Melatonin
- ☐ Restoril (Temazepam)
- ☐ Rozerem (Ramelteon)
- ☐ Silenor (Doxepin)
- ☐ Sonata (Zaleplon)
- ☐ Trazodone (Oleptro)
- ☐ Zolpimist (Zolpidem)

****

- ☐ Contrave (Naltrexone)
- ☐ Hetlioz (Tasimelteon)
- ☐ Mirapex (Pramipexole)
- ☐ Neupro Patch (Rotigotine)
- ☐ Nuvigil (Armodafinil)
- ☐ Provigil (Modafinil)
- ☐ Requip (Ropinirole)
- ☐ Wakix (Pitolisant)
- ☐ Xyrem (Sodium Oxybate)

****

- ☐ Adderall (Amphetamine/ Dextroamphetimine)
- ☐ Adzenys (Amphetamine)
- ☐ Concerta (Methylphenidate)
- ☐ Contrave (Bupropion/ Naltrexone)

☐ Cotempla (Methylphenidate)

☐ Daytrana (Methylphenidate)

☐ Dexedrine (Dextroamphetamine)

☐ Dyanavel (Amphetamine)

☐ Evekeo (Amphetamine Sulfate)

☐ Focalin (Dexmethylphenidate)

☐ Focalin XR

****

☐ Intuniv (Guanfacine)

☐ Metadate (Methylphenidate Hydrochloride)

☐ Metadate CR

☐ Methylin (Methylphenidate)

☐ Methylphenidate

☐ Mydayis (Dextroamphetamine Amphetamine)

☐ Phentermine

☐ Quillichew (Methylphenidate)

☐ Quillivant XR (Methylphenidate Hydrochloride)

☐ Ritalin (Methylphenidate)

☐ Saxenda (Liraglutide)

☐ Strattera (Atomoxetine)

☐ Vyvanse (Lisdexamfetamine)

☐ Zenzedi (Dextroamphetamine Sulfate)

****

☐ Ativan (Lorazepam)

☐ Buspar (Buspirone)

☐ Inderal (Propranolol)

☐ Klonopin (Clonazepam)

☐ Librium (Chlordiazepoxide)

☐ Niravam (Alprazolam)

☐ Valium (Diazepam)

☐ Vistaril (Hydroxyzine)

☐ Xanax (Alprazolam)

****

☐ Actiq (Fentanyl)

☐ Fentanyl (Abstral, Subsys)

☐ Hydrocodone

☐ Lortab (Hydrocodone)

☐ Methadone

☐ Morphine (Duramorph, Astramorph)

☐ Norco (Acetaminophen/ Hydrocodone)

☐ Nucynta (Tapentadol)

☐ Oxycodone (Roxicodone, Oxecta)

☐ OxyContin (Oxycodone)

☐ Percocet (Acetaminophen/ Oxycodone)

☐ Suboxone (Buprenorphine)

☐ Tramadol (ConZip, Ryzolt)

☐ Ultram (Tramadol)

Instructions:

1. Write the date, day of the week, type of day (work, school day off/vacation) on both graphs
2. Put the following: "C" for coffee, cola, or tea intake, "M" for medicine intake, "A" for alcohol, and "E" for exercise on bot
3. Put a line (I) when you go to bed - see example
4. Shade in the box when you think you went to sleep or took a nap on both graphs - see example

DAYTIME: (8:00 am - 8:00 pm)

Date	Day	Day Type	8 AM	9 AM	10 AM	11 AM	NOON	1 PM	2 PM	3 PM	4 PM	5 PM	6 PM	7 PM	8 PM
Example	MON	Vacation													

NIGHTTIME: (9:00 pm - 7:00 am)

Date	Day	Day Type	9 PM	10 PM	11 PM	12 PM	MIDNIGHT	1 AM	2 AM	3 AM	4 AM	5 AM	6 AM	7 AM
Example	MON	Vacation												

About the Author

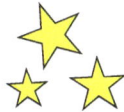

Dr. Debra Stultz is an author, professional speaker, and physician living in Huntington, WV. She is in private practice at Stultz Sleep & Behavioral Health. She is board-certified in psychiatry, sleep medicine, and behavioral sleep medicine. She graduated from Marshall University School of Medicine. She then completed her psychiatry residency and a child and adolescent psychiatry fellowship with West Virginia University School of Medicine – Charleston Division.

Her first book, *Wake Up Sleepy Head! Diagnosing, Understanding, and Navigating Narcolepsy*, addresses various causes of excessive daytime sleepiness with a focus on narcolepsy. She has authored numerous scientific articles and poster presentations. She is the editor of the "TMS Today" newsletter for the Clinical TMS Society. She is a member of The International Society for Sports Psychiatry with an interest in sleep and mental health in athletes.

She is a nationwide speaker on topics such as narcolepsy, insomnia, transcranial magnetic stimulation (TMS) for resistant depression, treating excessive daytime sleepiness, the treatment of obstructive sleep apnea associated with obesity, and various other health/ wellness topics.

She is passionate about teaching and educating others about the interaction between sleep disorders, psychiatric disorders, and other medical disorders. She has a special interest in transcranial magnetic stimulation (TMS) and the use of Spravato for resistant depression, sports psychiatry, head injuries, insomnia, and narcolepsy.

Dr. Stultz can be reached at (304) 733-5380.

For more information, visit Stultz Sleep & Behavioral Health at www.drdebrastultz.com

DR. DEBRA STULTZ

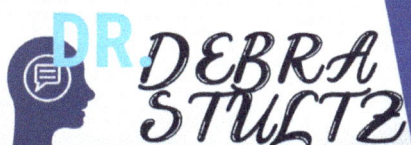

SPEAKER PRESENTATIONS

Dr. Stultz is an enthusiastic, sincere, inspiring, and motivating speaker to providers, patients, students, sleep fellows, residents, and therapists. She shares her 30+ years of experience as a Psychiatrist, Author, Internationally-known Speaker, and Sleep Physician.

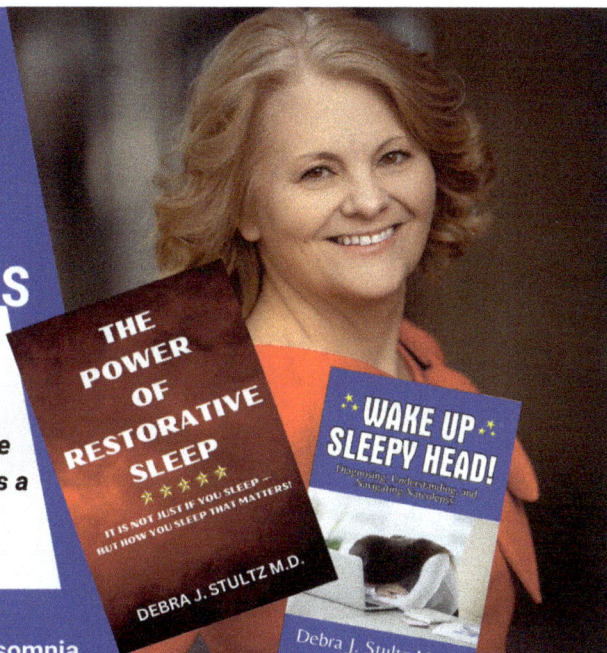

THE POWER OF RESTORATIVE SLEEP
IT IS NOT JUST IF YOU SLEEP – BUT HOW YOU SLEEP THAT MATTERS!
DEBRA J. STULTZ M.D.

WAKE UP SLEEPY HEAD!
Insomnia, Understanding, and Managing Sleepiness
Debra J. Stultz M.D.

✓ Narcolepsy & Idiopathic Hypersomnia
- Treatment and Diagnosis of Narcolepsy and other Causes of Hypersomnia
- Pharmacological Options, Behavioral Treatments and Family Interventions
- Pediatric, Adolescent, Adult, and Elderly Presentations of Narcolepsy

✓ Treatment-Resistant Depression
- Identifying All of the Pieces of the Puzzle Contributing to Resistant Depression
- New and Novel Treatments of Depression

✓ Transcranial Magnetic Stimulation
- Non-Medication Treatment for Depression, Migraines, and OCD
- Upcoming Indications for TMS Use in Substance Abuse, Pain, Strokes, etc.

✓ Diagnosing and Treating Sleep Disorders
- Comprehensive Evaluation and Diagnosis Contributing to Insomnia and Hypersomnia
- Pharmacologic and Behavioral Treatments of Insomnia and Other Sleep Disorders

Lectures can be provided in-person or online for events, such as conferences, promotional gatherings, seminars, and private events.

📞 (304) 733-5380

🌐 www.drdebrastultz.com

📍 52 Childers Rd., Barboursville, WV 25504

✉️ wvsleepdoc@outlook.com

Stultz Sleep
& Behavioral Health

215

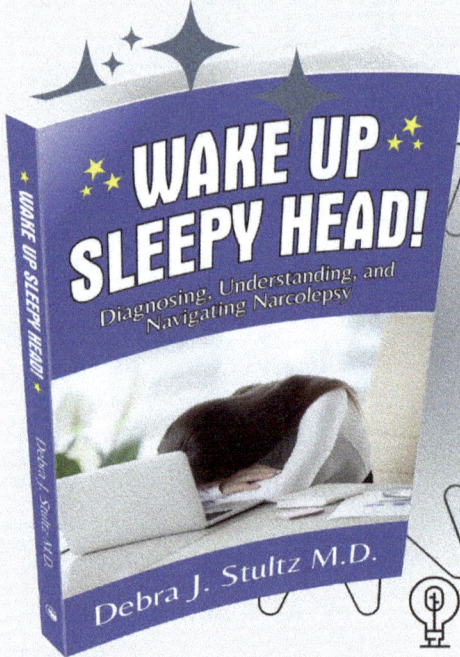

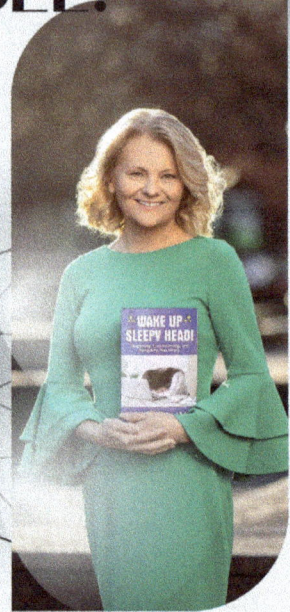

**If you find either of these books informative or enjoyable, it would be very valuable to me if you left a review on Amazon, Goodreads, my Facebook author page, or other book sites. Thank you!

Audio Versions of

The Power of Restorative Sleep

and

Wake Up Sleepy Head!

will be available at:

www.DrDebraStultz.com

Audible, Spotify, Apple Books, BAM, chirp, audiobooksnow, Google Play, and other fine audiobook online sites.

"Stop the Sleep Stealing" tip sheets and "Please Be Quiet! Shift Worker Fast Asleep" door hangers are also available at our website above.

www.ingramcontent.com/pod-product-compliance
Lightning Source LLC
Chambersburg PA
CBHW052111030426
42335CB00025B/2937